RESEARCH ADVANCES IN COMMUNICATION STUDIES

INTRODUCTION TO COMMUNICATION SCIENCES

RESEARCH ADVANCES IN COMMUNICATION STUDIES

Additional books and e-books in this series can be found on Nova's website under the Series tab.

RESEARCH ADVANCES IN COMMUNICATION STUDIES

INTRODUCTION TO COMMUNICATION SCIENCES

S. R. SAVITHRI

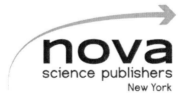

Copyright © 2019 by Nova Science Publishers, Inc.

All rights reserved. No part of this book may be reproduced, stored in a retrieval system or transmitted in any form or by any means: electronic, electrostatic, magnetic, tape, mechanical photocopying, recording or otherwise without the written permission of the Publisher.

We have partnered with Copyright Clearance Center to make it easy for you to obtain permissions to reuse content from this publication. Simply navigate to this publication's page on Nova's website and locate the "Get Permission" button below the title description. This button is linked directly to the title's permission page on copyright.com. Alternatively, you can visit copyright.com and search by title, ISBN, or ISSN.

For further questions about using the service on copyright.com, please contact:
Copyright Clearance Center
Phone: +1-(978) 750-8400   Fax: +1-(978) 750-4470   E-mail: info@copyright.com.

NOTICE TO THE READER

The Publisher has taken reasonable care in the preparation of this book, but makes no expressed or implied warranty of any kind and assumes no responsibility for any errors or omissions. No liability is assumed for incidental or consequential damages in connection with or arising out of information contained in this book. The Publisher shall not be liable for any special, consequential, or exemplary damages resulting, in whole or in part, from the readers' use of, or reliance upon, this material. Any parts of this book based on government reports are so indicated and copyright is claimed for those parts to the extent applicable to compilations of such works.

Independent verification should be sought for any data, advice or recommendations contained in this book. In addition, no responsibility is assumed by the Publisher for any injury and/or damage to persons or property arising from any methods, products, instructions, ideas or otherwise contained in this publication.

This publication is designed to provide accurate and authoritative information with regard to the subject matter covered herein. It is sold with the clear understanding that the Publisher is not engaged in rendering legal or any other professional services. If legal or any other expert assistance is required, the services of a competent person should be sought. FROM A DECLARATION OF PARTICIPANTS JOINTLY ADOPTED BY A COMMITTEE OF THE AMERICAN BAR ASSOCIATION AND A COMMITTEE OF PUBLISHERS.

Additional color graphics may be available in the e-book version of this book.

Library of Congress Cataloging-in-Publication Data

ISBN: 978-1-53616-209-7

Published by Nova Science Publishers, Inc. † New York

CONTENTS

List of Figures		vii
List of Tables		xiii
Preface		xv
Chapter 1	Speech, Language and Communication	1
Chapter 2	Bases of Speech and Language	49
Chapter 3	Sound Intensity and Concept of Decibel	141
Chapter 4	Audibility and Hearing	157
Chapter 5	Introduction to Speech-Language Pathology and Audiology	189
About the Author		249
Index of Names		251
Index of Terms		255
Related Nova Publications		259

LIST OF FIGURES

Figure 1.	Schematic diagram of respiratory system, the laryngeal system and the resonatory system	2
Figure 2.	Illustration of stream and puffs of air	3
Figure 3.	Illustration of pitch in child, man and woman	4
Figure 4.	Illustration of normal and hoarse voice	5
Figure 5.	Vocal tract structures	6
Figure 6.	Illustration of vocal tract structures in a tube	7
Figure 7.	Illustration of vowel production through water from hose pipe	9
Figure 8.	Analogy of a hose pipe for the production of stop consonant	10
Figure 9.	Analogy of a hose pipe for the production of fricatives	11
Figure 10.	Analogy of a hose pipe for the production of nasal continuants	12
Figure 11.	Forms of language	16
Figure 12.	Illustration of similarities of speech, language and communication	21

viii — *List of Figures*

Figure 13.	The speech chain	24
Figure 14.	Speech areas of cerebral hemisphere	52
Figure 15.	Larynx in an adult male	54
Figure 16.	Illustration of the function of vocal folds	55
Figure 17.	The resonatory system	56
Figure 18.	A sieve	56
Figure 19.	Illustration of the filters in the production of /g/ and /d/	57
Figure 20.	Tuning fork	59
Figure 21.	Motion of right prong of the tuning fork	59
Figure 22.	Curve tracing motion of tuning fork prong	60
Figure 23.	Tuning fork along with curve tracing motion	60
Figure 24.	Waves of frequencies 200 Hz, and 400 Hz	60
Figure 25.	Waveforms with different amplitudes	62
Figure 26.	Motion of a pendulum	63
Figure 27.	The displacement and velocity curves of pendulum bob	64
Figure 28.	Motion of point P on the circumference of a circle	65
Figure 29.	Graph of the sines of angles from 0^0 to 360^0	66
Figure 30.	Two sine waves with 90^0 difference of phase	67
Figure 31.	Two sine waves with 180^0 difference of phase	68
Figure 32.	Addition of two sine waves with 90^0 difference of phase	69
Figure 33.	(a) Addition of two sine waves with different frequencies, (b) addition of waveforms with 3 different frequencies	69

List of Figures

ix

Figure 34.	Displacement of a highly damped system	71
Figure 35.	Two waveforms with slightly different frequency and the beat produced by them	72
Figure 36.	Individual water particles moving up and down	73
Figure 37.	Propagation of a wave along a rope	74
Figure 38.	Illustration of a hammer hitting the table on the side	75
Figure 39.	Particle movement when a hammer is hit on the side of a table	75
Figure 40.	Longitudinal and transverse waves	76
Figure 41.	Particle motion in the path of a longitudinal wave	77
Figure 42.	Compression and rarefaction in a longitudinal wave created by vibration of tuning fork	78
Figure 43.	Wavelength represented by peak to peak or crest to crests or zero crossings	80
Figure 44.	Standing wave	82
Figure 45.	Different modes of vibration in a string	84
Figure 46.	Forced vibration of the table top in response to a tuning fork	85
Figure 47.	Resonance curves of two systems	87
Figure 48.	Multiple resonances of an air column in a jar	87
Figure 49.	Illustration of a sound spectrum	88
Figure 50.	Speech production as a filtering process	90
Figure 51.	The source and the filter in the vocal tract	90
Figure 52.	Schematic diagram of voice source (a) and waveform (b)	92
Figure 53.	Illustration of source spectrum	93

X   *List of Figures*

Figure 54.   Fundamental and harmonic partials
                   of the voice source   93

Figure 55.   A glottal waveform   94

Figure 56.   Opening and closing of the vocal folds   95

Figure 57.   Silence waveform   95

Figure 58.   Schematic diagram of a whispering sound (a)
                   and waveform (b)   96

Figure 59.   Schematic diagram of a frication (a)
                   and waveform (b)   98

Figure 60.   Illustration of a plosive production (a)
                   and waveform (b)   98

Figure 61.   Illustration of voice + noise source (a)
                   and waveform (b)   99

Figure 62.   Illustration of resonance   100

Figure 63.   Illustration of the first three resonances in a tube
                   closed at one end (R1 = First resonance,
                   R2 = Second resonance, R3 = Third resonance)   102

Figure 64.   Illustration of the first three resonances in
                   a tube open at one end (R1 = First resonance,
                   R2 = Second resonance, R3 = Third resonance)   103

Figure 65.   3-D shape – MRI image (a) cylindrical sections
                   (b) of vocal tract (Source: Internet)   104

Figure 66.   Illustration of filter   105

Figure 67.   Illustration of source, transfer function (TF)
                   and product   106

Figure 68.   Illustration of resonances in the vocal tract
                   (N = Node, A = antinode)   107

Figure 69.   Illustration of vocal tract as back and front cavity   107

List of Figures

Figure 70.	Illustration of source, transfer function and product in the production of vowel /a/	108
Figure 71.	Illustration of vocal tract configuration, source, transfer function and product in the production of vowel /i/	109
Figure 72.	Illustration of vocal tract configuration, source, transfer function and product in the production of vowel /u/	110
Figure 73.	Showing the articulatory positioning and area function for all three vowels	110
Figure 74.	Showing the formant frequencies arising out of the variable resonator – vocal tract – for three vowels	111
Figure 75.	A neuron with cell body, axon and dendrites	114
Figure 76.	Brodmann areas	118
Figure 77.	Lateral surface of cerebrum	121
Figure 78.	Superior view of the cerebral hemisphere	121
Figure 79.	Drawing of cerebellum	122
Figure 80.	Cross section of spinal cord	124
Figure 81.	Meninges	125
Figure 82.	Schematic diagram of the pyramidal system in speech production, and the cranial nerves responsible for the innervations of the muscles used in phonation, resonance, and articulation	128
Figure 83.	Parts of human ear	160
Figure 84.	Cross-section of a loop of the cochlea	163
Figure 85.	A typical psychometric function	169

xii   *List of Figures*

Figure 86.   A series of descending and ascending runs
                  in the method of limits   171

Figure 87.   Illustration of the method of adjustment   172

Figure 88.   Equal loudness contours   177

Figure 89.   Helmholtz resonator   208

Figure 90.   Visible speech   211

Figure 91.   The first Kymograph   212

Figure 92.   Voder demonstration at the World Fair, New York   213

Figure 93.   The sound spectrograph   214

Figure 94.   The Pattern Play Back   215

Figure 95.   An Electromyograph   215

Figure 96.   A Manometer   216

Figure 97.   A laryngeal mirror used by Manuel Garcia   217

Figure 98.   An Electroglottograph and the EGG signal
                  (Glottal enterprises)   218

Figure 99.   Electropalate and EPG   218

Figure 100.   ERP showing P1, N1, P2, and N2   219

LIST OF TABLES

Table 1.	Hindi alphabets in De:vana:gari script	13
Table 2.	Speech sound acquisition	26
Table 3.	Cranial nerves with their functions	51
Table 4.	Sines of angles from 0^0 to 90^0	66
Table 5.	Examples of sound power in Watts and sound power level in decibels from some sources	144
Table 6.	Intensity and the corresponding dB levels	153
Table 7.	Example of loudness in sone, along with sound pressure and SPL	179
Table 8.	A comparison of sone and phon	180
Table 9.	Threshold of pain and the corresponding sound pressure	182
Table 10.	Organization of phonemes in Sanskrit	208

PREFACE

The main theme of the book Introduction to Communication Sciences is to provide information on (a) communication, language, speech & their components in brief with illustrations, (b) production, characteristics and generation of sound in detail, (c) sound intensity and concept of decibel, (d) hearing mechanism, audibility and hearing, and (e) introduction to the field of speech-language pathology and audiology including historical aspects of these two fields in five chapters. It is primarily written for libraries and with an intention of helping students studying in the first year of the speech and hearing Bachelor's programme, master's students in Speech Pathology, research scholars, and faculty teaching Speech Pathology and Audiology. The book is different from others as it incorporates literature from ancient Sanskrit literature and includes several illustrations for ease of understanding. It *incorporates* definitions of speech, language, communication, and their components, functions of communication, normal development of speech & language, pre-requisites and factors affecting speech-language development, cultural and linguistic issues in communication; bi/multilingual issues. It *addresses* overview of speech production, speech mechanism, the acoustic theory of speech production, and bases of speech and language. In addition, the book *focuses* on acoustic energy and power, absolute and relative units and measurements, Bel and deciBel, sound pressure and decibel sound pressure levels, and characteristics and application of decibels. Hearing mechanism, audibility and hearing is also *dealt* with along with hearing range, procedures of estimating minimum audible levels, minimum audible pressure and field, reference equivalent threshold sound pressure levels and hearing levels, and other related issues. Finally, it *introduces* the historical aspects of the field of Speech-Language Pathology and Audiology, development of the field in global context, interdisciplinary nature of the field, development of instrumentation in the field, and scope of practice of the field. As historical aspects are dealt with, material from WWW were included and hence internet references were inevitable.

The course is required/hard core/discipline specific core course, and hence the proposed book would be used as a *primary text*. With its reader-friendly content and valuable online resources, *Introduction to Communication Sciences* is an ideal text for beginning speech pathology and audiology students and faculty.

Chapter 1

SPEECH, LANGUAGE AND COMMUNICATION

INTRODUCTION

Communication is essential for our day-to-day activities. All of us would have heard a baby crying. This is his/ her first communication with the world. When one says his/her name the tongue, lips move. This is communication through *speech*. All of us would have seen people using handshake (*gestures*) to greet others which is a means of communication. When one fills in an application or writes the test/examination s/he uses a script. Hence *writing* is also a means of communication. Therefore, one can express his ideas by speech, and other modes such as gestures and writing. Any means, vocal or other, of expressing or communicating thought or feelings is *language*.

Let us take a look into the speech system. Figure 1 shows the respiratory system, comprising of lungs and trachea; the laryngeal system comprising of the vocal folds, and the resonatory system comprising of the oral cavity and the nasal cavity, together called the vocal tract.

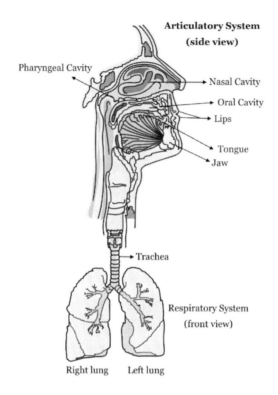

Figure 1. Schematic diagram of respiratory system, the laryngeal system and the resonatory system.

The expiratory air, noise, moves upwards and is impeded by the vocal folds that convert the air to sound, voice. The voice enters the vocal tract and is modified by the articulators, i.e., tongue, lips, teeth and roof of the mouth, into speech which is radiated through the lips.

1. Definitions of Speech, Language, Communication, and Their Components

1.1. Speech

Speech is the verbal mode of communication or it is communication through vocal or oral symbols. The basis of speech as already explained in the paragraph above is expiratory air. Hence, *speech is the sound produced by vocal folds and modified by the articulators*. It is also a mode of communication through conventional vocal or oral symbols. The components of speech are voice, articulation, fluency and prosody.

1.1.1. Voice

We already understood that the expiratory air, a stream of air which is inharmonic in nature, passes through the vocal folds situated in the larynx. The vocal folds vibrate or close and open alternately and at a fast rate. The stream of air is stopped when the vocal folds close and is allowed to pass through when they open. This stopping and passing of air assist in converting the stream of air, noise, into puffs of air, voice, which is harmonic in nature. This puff of air is termed voice or *voice is the sound produced primarily by the vibration of vocal folds. Some define voice as a sound produced by the vibration of vocal folds and modified by the articulators.* This can be compared to persons passing through a wicket gate. Assume a queue of people standing behind the wicket gate which can be compared to the stream of expiratory air or noise. As the wicket gate allows one person at a time the queue is converted to single persons that can be compared to puffs of air. Figure 2 illustrates stream and puffs of air.

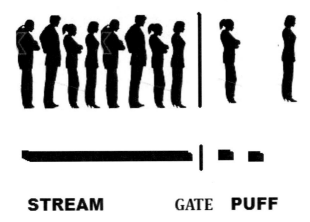

Figure 2. Illustration of stream and puffs of air.

1.1.2. Components of Voice

Pitch, loudness, and quality are the components of voice. *Pitch* is a perceptual correlate of frequency. Frequency refers to the number of vibrations per unit time and in this context refers to the vibrations of the vocal folds. We hear a pitch as high when the vibrations are more and low when the vibrations are low. All of have heard a child, a man and a woman speaking, and we understand that a child has a shrill voice, a man has a low voice and the voice of a women is in between. This component is pitch. A child has a high pitch, a man low pitch and a woman has a medium pitch. The vocal fold of a child vibrates at a rate of 300-400 times per second, and hence is perceived as high pitch. In men, the vibration is at a rate of 80-180 times per second and is perceived as low pitch. The vibration is around 180-280 times per second in woman. Pitch depends on age and gender, and is higher in children & lower in adults, and is higher in males compared to females. Figure 3 is an illustration of pitch in child, man and woman.

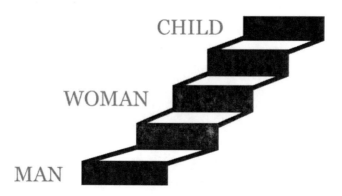

Figure 3. Illustration of pitch in child, man and woman.

Loudness is another component of voice. It is a perceptual correlate of intensity. When we speak to someone nearby, we speak in a soft voice and when calling someone far away, loud voice is used. A loud voice requires more expiratory air compared to a soft voice. *Quality* is another component which is a perceptual correlate of spectra. Voce qualities include breathy, harsh, hoarse, nasal etc. A breathy voice occurs when the air is passing through the open vocal folds or when the vocal folds are not completely closing or not adducting sufficiently and is presumed to have inadequate breath support. Harsh quality is when the vocal folds are over adducted, or the closure is fast. Hoarse is a combination of breathy and harsh qualities. Sometimes because of structural or functional problems the velopharyngeal port is open and the expiratory air passes through the nasal cavity instead of channelizing through the oral cavity resulting in nasal voice. In the production of /n/, /m/ etc. the air should be channelized through the nasal cavity. Nevertheless, one would have experienced a denasal voice when s/he has cold when the air is not channelized through the nasal cavity. Figure 4 is an illustration of normal and hoarse voice.

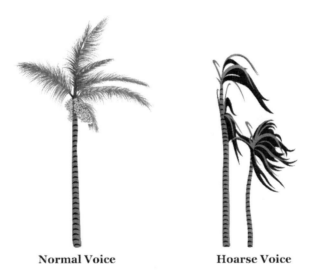

Normal Voice   **Hoarse Voice**

Figure 4. Illustration of normal and hoarse voice.

1.2. Articulation

Tongue, teeth, lips and roof of the mouth move in various ways when we speak. The word articulation in speech refers to the movement of articulators to produce speech sounds. Various places and manners of articulation are assumed by the articulators to produce speech sounds.

1.2.1. Oral Structure

The places of articulation from lip end includes bilabial, labio-dental, dental, alveolar, retroflex, palatal, velar, uvular, pharyngeal and glottal. Understanding of the oral structure is essential in understanding various places of articulation. Figure 5 shows the vocal tract structures and Figure 6 shows the same when the vocal tract is pulled and assumed as a tube.

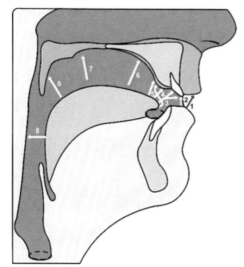

1) Lips
2) Teeth
3) Teeth
4) Alveolar ridge
5) Post-alveolus (hard palate)
6) Palate
7) Velum
8) Uvula
9) Pharynx

Source: http:// en.wikipedia.org/ wiki/ Place_of_articulation.

Figure 5. Vocal tract structures.

The *vocal tract* is divided into the *nasal cavity* (within the nose) and the *oral cavity* (the pharynx and mouth). The length of the vocal cavity (from the larynx to the lips/nostrils) is about 17 cm and that of the nasal cavity is about 12 cm in adult male. Some parts of the oral cavity can be used to produce sounds and are called *articulators*. Some articulators are movable (for example tongue) and are called active articulators; some are fixed (for example hard palate) and are called passive articulators. Generally, speech sounds are produced with at least one active and one passive articulator.

The *lips* are fleshy folds consisting of tissue, blood vessels, glands, nerves and muscle.

Speech, Language and Communication

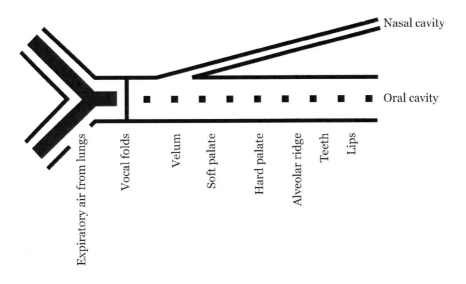

Figure 6. Illustration of vocal tract structures in a tube.

The *tongue* is the most mobile articulator and can move both vertically and laterally. The parts of the tongue are root, blade and tip. Immediately behind the upper teeth ridge is the *alveolus*, also called *alveolar ridge*, which is the projecting bony protrusion. When the tip of the tongue contacts the alveolar ridge to produce a sound, the resultant is said to be in the alveolar place of articulation.

The *hard palate* forms the roof of the mouth. This is a bony structure which lies just behind the alveolus. When the tip of the tongue touches the hard palate, the resultant sound is said to be in palatal place of articulation.

The *velum* or *soft palate* is composed of muscle fibers, tissue, blood vessels, nerves, and glands. It separates the oral cavity from the nasal cavity. By rising of the velum, it is pressed against the posterior wall of the pharynx and prevents air from going through the nose. This is essential for the production of oral sounds. When it is lowered, air passes through both the nose and mouth. Sounds articulated in this position are said to be in the velar place of articulation.

The *uvula* is the extension of the soft palate and is a small flap of tissue that hangs in the back of the mouth. Sounds articulated with the back of the tongue and the uvula are called uvular.

8 *S. R. Savithri*

The *epiglottis* is a leaf- like cartilage which is attached to the anterior part of the thyroid cartilage, and to the root of the tongue. It prevents food from entering the trachea by covering the entrance to the larynx during swallowing.

The *pharynx* is a funnel-shaped muscle tube of 8-12 cm in length. It stretches from the larynx and esophagus, the epiglottis and the root of the tongue, to the area in the back of the velum. The pharyngeal cavity is divided into three parts - the oropharynx that is at the back of the mouth and covers the area between the root of the tongue and the velum; the nasopharynx that is situated opposite to the entry to the nasal cavity, and the laryngopharynx -. The length, volume, and shape of the pharynx can be modified by the movement of the back of the tongue, the action of the muscles surrounding the pharynx, and the position of the velum. When it is raised, the nasopharynx is blocked.

The nose or *nasal cavity* has two parts – i.e., the nostrils – connected by a central bone known as the septum. The roof of the nasal cavity is very narrow, while the floor is smooth and relatively wide. The side walls are extremely irregular. At the back, it leads into the nasopharynx. The main functions of nose are the humidification and heating of air during respiration. It also acts as a filter and nasal sounds are produced when the air is channelized through nose.

1.2.2. Place of Articulation

Having now seen the oral structures we shall learn about the places of articulation. The sounds /p/, /b/, and /m/ are produced by moving lips together and this is called *bilabial* place of articulation. *Labio-dental* refers to the place when the lower lip moves towards the upper teeth as in the production of /f/ and /v/. *Dental* is the place of articulation when the tip of the tongue is moving towards the teeth as in the production of /t/, /d/, /n/, and /s/. *Alveolar* refers to the place of articulation when the tip of the tongue is moving towards the alveolar ridge and *retroflex* is when the tip of the tongue curls back and moves towards the palate as in the production of /t./, /d./, /n./ and /s./. Similarly, *palatal* is the place of the articulation when the mid of the tongue is moving towards the soft palate as in the production of

/c/, /j/, /n~/, & /ʃ/ and *velar* is when the back of the tongue moves towards the velum as in /k/, /g/, /n /; *Uvular* and *pharyngeal* are when the back of the tongue moves towards uvula and pharynx, respectively. *Glottal* place refers to the space between the vocal folds and the sound produced at glottal place of articulation is /h/.

1.2.3. Manner of Articulation

Manners of articulation refer to the way constrictions are formed in the vocal tract. In the production of /a/, /i/, /u/, /e/, and /o/, the articulators are moving towards the place of articulation, but are not completely contacting the place. The oral tract is almost open. Wide constriction area is observed between the articulator and the place of articulation and such a manner is referred to as *vowel*. The nasal tract is closed most of the time. None the less some languages have nasalized vowels Thus vowels are speech sounds produced by open oral tract and are used in all languages of the world. One can compare a vowel to water flowing through a hosepipe which is illustrated in Figure 7.

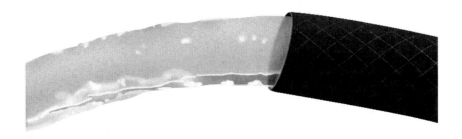

Figure 7. Illustration of vowel production through water from hose pipe.

Speech sounds other than vowels are called *consonants*. Consonants have different manners. Speech sounds such as /k/, /g/, /t /, /d /, /t/, /d/, /p/, and /b/ are produced with the articulator completely contacting the place of articulation thus closing the oral tract and hence the constriction area between the articulator and the place of articulation is zero. In such a condition, the air is held behind the articulator till the pressure is built in the oral tract and then is released. Such a manner is termed stop and the speech sounds produced by complete closure of the oral tract are called *stop consonants*. Stop consonants are available in most of the world's languages. One can again think of an analogy of a hosepipe by turning the water on and holding the finger blocking the water for some time. Take out the finger after some time and observe that a bump of water flows out. This is equivalent to a stop consonant. One can also think of a snap of a finger or eye blink. Thus, *stop consonants are speech sounds produced by closing the oral tract, building pressure behind it, and releasing the pressure by opening the articulator*. Figure 8 is an analogy for production of stop consonants.

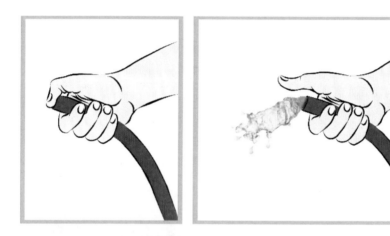

Figure 8. Analogy of a hose pipe for the production of stop consonant.

Some languages have speech sounds /c/ and /j/. These are essentially produced in the same way as stop consonants. But the articulatory release is different. The mid of the tongue lifts and contacts the palate, which is like a dome. Therefore, it takes longer time for the tongue to reach the palate and come back to the original position. Thus, the release of articulator is slow. These speech sounds are called *affricates*.

In the production of /s/, /h/, /s̪/ and /ʃ/, you can feel the air when you keep your finger in front of lips. In the production of such sounds, the tongue is lifted; but it doesn't contact the articulator completely and stop the air. There is a small constriction between the tongue and the articulator. The expiratory air when passing through this small constriction jets out at high pressure. These speech sounds are called *fricatives*. Fricatives are not many

Speech, Language and Communication

in Indian languages. The most common fricatives are /s/, and /h/. Again, one can think of the analogy of a hosepipe. Hold your finger at the end of the pipe to water plants at a distance and observe that the water jets out with high pressure. A whistle sound is produced in the same manner. Thus, *fricatives are speech sounds produced with a narrow constriction in the oral tract*. Figure 9 is an analogy for the production of a fricative.

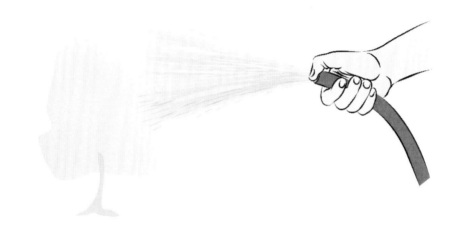

Figure 9. Analogy of a hose pipe for the production of fricatives.

Vowels, stop consonants, affricates and fricatives are produced with the velopharyngeal port closed, blocking the air to the nasal tract. There are some speech sounds that are produced with the velopharyngeal port open; for example, /m/, /n/ /n./ etc. In the production of such speech sounds, the air is channelized through the nasal tract, as the velopharyngeal port is open. The articulator completely closes the oral tract. Such speech sounds are called *nasal continuants*. Nasal continuants are used in most of the world's languages. An altogether different mechanism is used in producing nasal continuants. They are called continuants because one can prolong them, which is not possible with stop consonants. Thus, *nasal continuants are speech sounds produced with closed oral tract and open nasal tract*. Figure 10 is an analogy for the production of nasal continuants.

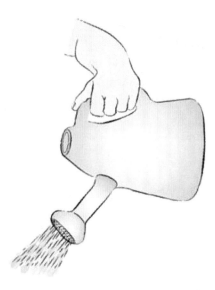

Figure 10. Analogy of a hose pipe for the production of nasal continuants.

Several other speech sounds are used in our languages. Some of these are combinations of two vowels; for example, /ai/, /au/. They are called *diphthongs*. /y/ and /v/ are also combinations of two vowels. /y/ is a combination of /i/ and /a/; /v/ is a combination of /u/ and /a/. In the production of diphthong /ai/, one can clearly hear both the vowels; but in the production of /y/ one can't. In a diphthong, the articulator moves slowly from one vowel to another; but in /y/, or /v/ the articulator moves fast from one vowel to another. Therefore, /y/ and /v/ are also called *glides*.

Assume a drone and imagine an upside drone in the oral tract. The middle part of the oral tract is closed, and the lateral sides are open. In such a vocal tract configuration, air passes through the sides of the tongue. These speech sounds are termed *laterals*. /l/ and /l̯/ are examples of laterals. Thus, *laterals are produced by blocking the oral tract in the middle and channelizing the air from the lateral sides.*

When one is imitating the sound of a car or a bus, the tip of the tongue is repeatedly contacting the palate. /r/ is produced in a similar manner and is called a *trill*. *A trill is a speech sound produced by repeated contacts of the articulator with the place of articulation.*

Speech, Language and Communication

13

Table 1. Hindi alphabets in De:vana:gari script

स्वर / Vowels

अ	आ	इ	ई	उ	ऊ	ऋ	ॠ	ए	ओ
a	a:	i	i:	u	u:	r̩	r̩:	e:	o:

संयुक्त स्वर/ द्विस्वर / Diphthongs

ऐ	औ
ai	au

घोष व्यंजन / Stop Consonants

क	ख	ग	घ
k	kh	g	gh

ट	ठ	ड	ढ़
t̩	t̩h	ḍ	ḍh

त	थ	द	ध
t	th	d	dh

प	फ	ब	भ
p	ph	b	bh

नासिक्य व्यंजन / Nasal Consonants

ङ	ण	न	म	ञ
n˙	ṇ	n	m	ñ

संघर्षी ध्वनियाँ / Fricatives

स	श	ष		ह
s	ś	ṣ		h

स्पर्श संघर्षी ध्वनियाँ / Affricates

च	छ	ज	झ
c	ch	j	jh

कंपित स्वर / Trill

र
r

पार्श्विक / Lateral

ल
l

श्रुति / Glides

य	व
y	v

14   S. R. Savithri

Further, there are distinctions of speech sounds in terms of voicing. For example, when you are saying vowel /a/, the vocal folds are vibrating; but it doesn't when you say /p/. Speech sounds, in the production of which vocal folds are vibrating are termed voiced and those which does not have vocal fold vibration are termed unvoiced. Also, some languages have speech sounds like /p/ and /ph/. /p/ uses less expiratory air compared to /ph/. Such speech sounds are termed unaspirated and speech sounds that relatively use more expiratory air are termed aspirated.

Thus, speech sounds can be classified as vowels and consonants and consonants have various manners, voicing and aspiration. It is very easy to remember these manners if you look at the script of your language. Hindi alphabets in De:vana:gari script is provided along with manner of articulation in Table 1. One can remember the various manners of speech sounds by studying the table. The principle is that the alphabets are arranged as per the manner. Open sounds are followed with closed sounds. The place of articulation moves from back to front in all manners of articulation. Whenever there is a distinction of voicing, voiced sounds follow unvoiced speech sounds. Aspirated speech sounds follow unaspirated, in case of a distinction between aspirated and unaspirated.

1.3. Fluency

Fluency is the continuous, effortless speech at a fast rate of speech (Starkweather, 1987). The parameters of fluency are continuity, effort and rate. Speech should be continuous for one to understand. Breaking the word in between, having pauses, repetitions of speech sounds/ words/ phrases/sentences, unwanted words not suitable for the sentence makes a sentence discontinuous. Therefore, *continuity* in speech is when the speech is devoid of repetitions, hesitations, pauses, false starts and parenthetical remarks. During speech there is *mental and muscular effort.* Mental effort refers to the coding in speech areas of the brain and muscular effort refers to the efforts of respiratory, laryngeal, and articulatory muscles. All these are to be timed and any mistiming will result in production of unwanted speech

Speech, Language and Communication   15

sound. For example, if one intends to produce the word /speech/, the speech sounds /s/, /p/, /I/, and /c/ have to be coded in such a way that they are approached in a serial manner and the nerve impulses reach the concerned muscle. Consider an instance when the oral tract is completely closed instead of a small constriction for the production of /s/. This would result in the production of /t/. Hence mental and muscular effort and timing is essential for the production of fluent speech. If, in a sentence, one word is spoken per 30 minutes it is difficult for the listener to understand it, for the simple reason that the rate of speech is extremely slow. The normal *rate* of speech is about 80-180 words per minute. Thus, the parameters of fluency are continuity, effort and rate. Disorders of fluency are stuttering and cluttering.

1.4. Prosody

Prosody is often not included as a component of speech. Prosody or suprasegmental refer to intonation, stress, rhythm, and pause. *Intonation* is the variation in pitch in the production of a phrase or a sentence. Such variations are essential without which speech would sound monotonous. *Stress* refers to extra effort on a syllable or a word. For example, in the sentence [Get me the RED book], the word /red/ can be stressed to negate books of other colors. *Rhythm* is a repeated movement. While the rhythm in poetry is regular it is not so regular in speech. *Pause* is a silence used between phrases, an important word, between sentences etc. For example, in the sentence [the University of Delhi was established in the year 1967 to provide quality education in the field of science, commerce, law, arts, and education], one pauses at several words like after 1967, science, commerce, law, arts, education. Pause is used to take breath, to inform the listener that something important is coming up and the sentence is complete etc. Intonation, stress and rhythm are superimposed on words and hence are called suprasegmental features.

2. LANGUAGE

Language is also a mode of communication and these modes include speech, writing, and gesture. Therefore, *language is a means, vocal or other, of expressing or communicating thought or feeling*. Figure 11 depicts the various forms of language.

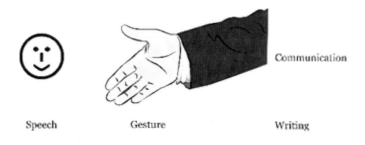

Figure 11. Forms of language.

2.1. Components of Language

Phonology, semantics, syntax, and pragmatics are components of language. The study of phonemes or speech sounds is termed *phonology*. A word is made by combining a set of phonemes. However, the order of the phonemes is important in creating a word. For example, if /s/, /p/, /i/, and /c/ are ordered serially it makes a meaningful word /speech/. However, the same phones ordered as /c/, /s/, /i/, and /p/, is not meaningful.

A relation between a word and meaning is created by the users of a language. For example, upon hearing the word /bus/ one remembers a vehicle. The meaning associated with this word is arbitrary but without a consensus on the meaning of a word, we can't communicate. Hence each word has a meaning. One can create a new language by assigning meanings to words. For example, assume that the following are the words/ symbols one has created in making a new language, in which each object is represented with a word by a group of people.

Speech, Language and Communication 17

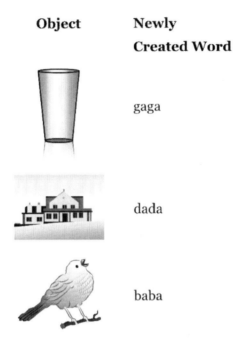

Object	Newly Created Word
(glass)	gaga
(house)	dada
(bird)	baba

If the same group of people practice this association between object and word, after some time when one says /gaga/, it will be associated with glass. Therefore, meaning of a word is learnt through exposure.

Language can be verbal or nonverbal, and gesture and writing are nonverbal modes of language. A group of people can arbitrarily assign some gestures to alphabets of a language. Imagine that the following gestures represent alphabets.

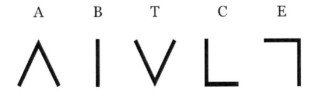

When they practice this, and they see | ∧∨ it is understood as /bat/ and ∧ L ⊓ is understood as /ace/. This study of relationship between word and meaning is called *semantics*.

18   *S. R. Savithri*

In running speech usually, you have a sentence and the words in a sentence should be interrelated. A combination of unrelated words like [tree box plate house] is meaningless, though each word has meaning. Together they don't give any meaning. On the other hand, a combination of words like [Rama killed Ravana] is meaningful, because, the words in this sentence are interrelated. The word 'Rama', subject, is associated with the word 'kill'; the word 'kill' is associated with the word 'Ravana', the object of the action killing and 'ed' in the word 'killed' indicates past tense. Hence this sentence is a combination of interrelated words to give meaning. The study of relationship between words is called *syntax*.

All of us have heard children speaking and imitating adults. Read the following paragraphs.

> "Prakash, Vijay's father, was working in an office. His boss used to shout at everyone in the office. All workers used to call him *Tughluk*. Prakash also used to refer to his boss at home as *Tughluk*. Once, Prakash invited his boss home for a party and he told Vijay not to speak the word *Tughluk* in front of his boss. Prakash's boss came home, and Vijay was standing behind the door at that time. He slowly came towards Prakash's boss. Prakash said 'Vijay, come greet uncle'. Vijay said 'Papa, is this the person whom you call *Tughluk*? I will see his anger and go'. Prakash's boss turned red."

We understand that Vijay doesn't know that he should not speak like this in front of his father's boss.

"Vijay's house was very nice, and his mother Sheela kept the house very neat and tidy. Once Vijay broke a glass. Sheela said 'Vijay! That is bad. Why did you break the glass? Some days later Sheela's friend Vijaya came home. Sheela gave her breakfast and milk. Unfortunately, the glass fell down and broke. Immediately Vijay said 'Aunty! That is bad. Why did you break the glass? Sheela was embarrassed.

Again, Vijay doesn't know that speaking with children and adults are different. The way you speak will be different when you speak the same matter with a child, your friend and an authority. For example, with a child you will speak 'baby come for lunch'; with a friend you will speak 'let us

Speech, Language and Communication 19

go for lunch' and with an authority you will speak 'may I request you to come for lunch? Thus, socially, you have different ways of speaking, the study of which is referred to as *pragmatics*. *Thus, the components of language are phonology, semantics, syntax, and pragmatics.*

3. COMMUNICATION

Communication is the process of transferring ideas, thoughts, feelings or opinions by means of signs, signals, and symbols expressed consciously or unconsciously from one to another. During speech there is a speaker and a listener, and the speaker is transferring the information to the listener through speech; similarly, the gesture, signs and signals are understood by the viewer and script is understood by the reader. Thus, two persons are essential in communication - one who provides information and others who receive the information - or a speaker, and a listener/s. Without two persons communication is impossible. Nevertheless, we communicate to ourselves often.

Components of communication include (a) context, (b) sender/ encoder/source, (c) message, (d) medium/ channel, (e) receiver/decoder, (f) effect, and (g) feedback. Every message usually commences with a context which consist of different aspects like country, culture, organization etc. It can also include external stimulus, the source of which may be letter, memo, telephone call, fax, note, email, meeting, and even a casual conversation. The external stimuli motivate one to respond which may be oral or written. Internal stimuli are also involved which includes opinion, attitude, likes, dislikes, emotions, experience, education and confidence. All these have complex influence on the way one communicates his ideas. Sender or encoder or source is one who is sending the message. In oral communication it is the speaker and in written communication the writer. The sender may use combination of words, symbols, graphs, pictures to convey his message to the receiver. Message refers to the information that is transmitted from the sender to the receiver. The sender should decide the content, information, and points of the message while considering the receiver. Medium is the channel through which the sender is communicating his message to the receiver. The medium may be sound (speech), print, electronic or it may be some person and it depends on the relationship between the sender and the receiver. The person to whom the message is sent is the receiver or decoder. He may be a listener (in case the media is speech), or a reader (in case the media is writing). Effect is the change in the behavior of the receiver in response to the message. The response or reaction of the receiver, to a message, is called feedback, which may also be oral or written, an action or silence. Feedback is very important component of communication as communication is effective only when a feedback is received.

4. DISTINCTIONS, SIMILARITIES AND FUNCTIONS OF COMMUNICATION, SPEECH AND LANGUAGE

4.1. Distinctions of Communication, Speech, and Language

Having defined communication as transferring ideas, thoughts, feelings or opinions by means of signs, signals, and symbols expressed consciously or unconsciously from one to another, one can communicate without language and speech. For example, you can smile, use facial expressions to communicate. Language is one means of communication. One can have normal speech and language but may have difficulty in communicating as in Autism Spectrum Disorder.

Having defined language as a means, vocal or other, of expressing or communicating thought or feeling, one can have language without speech. For example, one can use writing to communicate. Speech is verbal language and one means of communication.

4.2. Similarities of Communication, Speech, and Language

Speech can be thought as a sub-set of language and language can be thought of a sub-set of communication. So, communication is a wide concept encompassing speech, language, facial expressions, and others. Figure 12 illustrates the similarities of speech, language and communication.

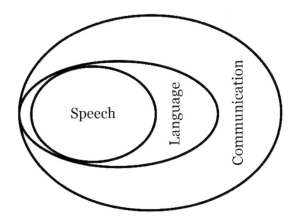

Figure 12. Illustration of similarities of speech, language and communication.

5. SPEECH AS AN OVERLAID FUNCTION

Several systems of the body are involved in speech production. These include nervous system, respiratory system, phonatory system, and articulatory or resonatory system. Of these, nervous system is a central system and the others are peripheral. A desire to speak activates the *nervous system*, which with the help of some areas in parietal & frontal lobes, organize the words and convert it into neural impulses through various nerves, or generate and send commands to the other systems of speech production. The nervous system issues command to respiratory, laryngeal, and articulatory or resonatory systems.

The *respiratory system* has two lungs at one end and the nostrils at the other end. The two lungs join together to form a tube called trachea. The trachea runs from lungs to throat. From there it enters the larynx and divides into mouth (oral tract) and nose (nasal tract). The function of the respiratory system is respiration, which is the process of breathing for *gas exchange*. It has two phases- inspiration and expiration -. Air is breathed in during inspiration through the nose where it is filtered and sent to lungs. On reaching the lungs Oxygen is separated from air. Carbon Dioxide (CO_2) is breathed out during expiration. Thus, the respiratory system acts like a pump by pushing the air in and pumping out the air. Lungs expand during inspiration and contract during expiration. We inspire about 60 times per second. The lungs can be compared to a rubber band or a harmonium. Therefore, the primary function of respiratory system is gas exchange. None the less, *secondarily* it is used for speech production. In quiet respiration, the air is breathed in and out through the nose. But, in speech production, expiration can be through mouth or nose. In quiet breathing, inspiration and expiration share 50% each. But inspiration is shorter, and expiration is longer for speech purposes. The respiratory system supplies energy or AIR for speech which has a pressure of about 5-8 cm of H_2O. Therefore, *speech production is a superimposed function of the respiratory system.*

The *laryngeal system* consists of the larynx or the voice box, which is situated in between the trachea and the oral tract. The larynx is made up of a bone, cartilages and muscles and is suspended in the neck. The most important part of the larynx is vocal folds. The vocal folds act like a soldier guarding the border. They protect the lungs from entering food by closing and this is the basic function of vocal folds. They also push the dust/ unwanted particles out in the inspiratory air by cough or sneeze. Therefore, the *primary function of the vocal folds is protective in nature*. However, they also help in speech production as a secondary function. They vibrate when the air passes through them or open and close and convert it to voice. The length of the vocal folds is about 10-17 mm. The length changes with age and gender. It is short in children and long in adults. These small vocal folds can produce amazing voice. The vocal folds can vibrate anywhere between 80 times per second to 800 times per second. T*hus, voicing is a secondary function of the laryngeal system.*

Speech, Language and Communication   23

The *resonatory system* includes (a) pharynx, (b) the oral cavity, and (c) the nasal cavity with the velopharyngeal port separating the oral cavity from the nasal cavity. The organs in the oral cavity are used for chewing and sending the food bolus to pharynx from where it is pushed to the digestive tract. *The primary function of the nasal tract is filtering the inspiratory air and sending it to lungs.* Nevertheless, the resonatory system also helps in speech production. The oral cavity and the nasal cavity act like filters and selectively filter the laryngeal sound to produce various speech sounds depending on the placement of articulators. Hence, *speech production is an overlaid function of the resonatory system.*

Having learnt the functions of different systems, one understands that the basic function of the respiratory system is respiration; that of the laryngeal system is protection; that of the articulatory system is chewing or mastication. They are not meant for speech production. But it is remarkable that they take on additional functions of speech production. Therefore, *speech is called an overlaid function.*

6. SPEECH CHAIN

The speech chain is a description of the stages in speech communication when a message is transferred from the speaker to the listener linguistically. The speaker has a thought which he encodes into a sequence of articulatory gestures. This process is termed articulatory planning and execution. The articulatory gestures generate speech sounds (speech acoustics) which reach the ears of the listener, and the speaker also for feedback. The transmission of speech sound is termed acoustics. The acoustic information passes through the external ear to the middle ear where it is converted to mechanical energy and further reaches the inner ear and is processed into a neural code (hearing). This neural code is decoded in the brain of the listener to extract the meaning of the utterance, and the intention of the act of communication (speech perception).

Auditory feedback is critical when one is learning to speak. The feedback provides knowledge of how different articulations create different sounds. Children who are born with hearing impairment have difficulty in learning to speak compared to hearing children. The quality and intelligibility of our speech production can be monitored by auditory feedback. The speech of adults who acquire hearing loss can have speech problems as they are unable to monitor their own articulation. The visual information, that is the movements of the various articulators in the mouth of the speaker, can also be useful to the listener, especially in poor listening environment. Under such circumstances, the listener tries to lip read the speaker.

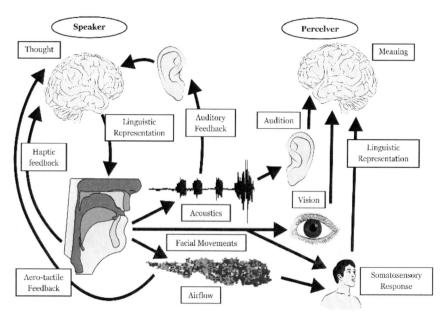

Source: https://www.google.com/search?q=speech+chain&tbm=isch&source=univ&sa=X&ved=2ahUKEwi1tPX519HiAhUBN48KHceJCSAQsAR6BAgDEAE&biw=1440&bih=735#imgrc=oAsoQ9QrLKhxyM.

Figure 13. The speech chain.

There are some processing stages and the knowledge that speakers and listeners use at each stage. These processes and the knowledge include (a) decision of how to achieve effect in listener (word knowledge), (b) generating utterances that match the intended meaning (knowledge of

Speech, Language and Communication 25

meaning and grammar), (c) use appropriate prosody (knowledge of prosody), (d) execute motor plan for articulatory movement (knowledge of articulatory consequences of articulation), in the listener (e) listening to the utterances, recovering the meaning and intentions of the speaker. Figure 13 depicts the speech chain.

7. NORMAL DEVELOPMENT OF SPEECH AND LANGUAGE

7.1. Normal Development of Speech Sounds

As discussed earlier, speech is a verbal means of communicating or conveying meaning and is a result of specific motor behaviors. Therefore, speech requires precise neuromuscular coordination. As the child matures, he gains increasing control of the speech mechanism and is able to produce or articulate sounds more effectively. Although he gains a large amount of motor control in first year, the child does not achieve adult like stability until mid-childhood. Speech starts with the *birth cry*. Between the birth and one month, the child has reflexive behaviors like sucking and swallowing, non-differentiated crying, vegetative sounds (burps, gurgle sounds) and noises. Between 2-3 months, s/he shows *cooing* behavior which includes movement of some articulators, production of velar/ back consonants and mid vowels. Greater control of tongue during 4-6 months results in prolonged strings of sounds, more lip or labial sounds, and the child starts experimenting with sounds. The stage is termed *babbling*. 6-10 months is a stage of *reduplicated babbling/ lalling*, where the child has repetitive syllable production, increased lip control, production of labial, alveolar and plosives /p/, /b/, /t/, /d/, nasals, /j/, but not yet fully formed. The *first word* appears between 11-14 months. The child uses phonetically consistent forms, elevates tongue tip, has variegated babbling, intonational patterns, understands sound-meaning relationships, predominantly uses /m, w, b, p/. The first word primarily consists of CV (pa), VC (am), or CVCV (mama). By 2 years of age, the child acquires phonemes /p/, /h/, /w/, /m/, /n/, /b/, /k/, /g/. By 3 years of age, the child acquires /d/, /f/, /j/, /t/, /n/, /s/; by 4 years /v/, /ʃ/, /tʃ/, /z/; by 5 years

26   *S. R. Savithri*

/r/, /l/, /dz/, /th/ and by 6-8 years /Z/, consonant blends. Development of speech sounds is summarized in Table 2.

Table 2. Speech sound acquisition

Sl. No.	Age	Stage	Speech
1	0-1 month	New born	Reflexive behavior like sucking and swallowing, non-differentiated crying, vegetative sounds (burps, gurgle sounds) and noises.
2	2-3 months	Cooing	Definite stop and start to oral movement, velar to uvular closure or near closure, back consonants and back and middle vowels with incomplete resonance.
3	4-6 months	Babbling	Greater independent control of tongue, prolonged strings of sounds, more lip or labial sounds, experiments with sounds.
4	6-10 months	Reduplication babbling	Repetitive syllable production, increased lip control, labial, alveolar and plosives /p/, /b/, /t/, /d/, nasals, /j/, but not fully formed.
5	11-14 months	Phonetically consistent forms and first words.	Elevates tongue tip, variegated babbling, intonational patterns, phonetically consistent forms, sound-meaning relationships, predominance of /m, w, b, p/, first words primarily CV (pa), VC (am), CVCV (mama).
6	2 years		Acquires simple words
7	3 years		Acquires /d, f, j, t, n, s/.
8	4 years		Acquires /v, ʃ, tʃ, z/
9	5 years		Acquires /r, l, dz, th/
10	6-8 years		Acquires /Z/, consonant blends.

7.1.1. Development of Fluency

The ability to speak fluently is a skill that develops as children grow. All children, between the ages of 2 and 6, occasionally hesitate as they begin to put sounds, words, and sentences together. The child may exhibit word or phrase *repetitions*, repeat part-words revise sentences, use filled *pauses* (such as mm, aa etc.), silent pauses, hesitate to speak, use *false starts* and *parenthetical remarks*. Example of repitition is [I I I will go to school]. Filled pauses will be [I want mm mm ball]. An example of false start is [That is a *blue no red* bus], parenthetical remarks are expressions like you mean, I know etc. which are meaningful but irrelevant for the situation. These are termed disfluencies and are normal. Boys have been reported to have more disfluencies than girls. Never the less they come out of the disfluencies as

Speech, Language and Communication 27

they grow. In early stages children use more of repetitions and pauses but use more sophisticated disfluencies such as false starts and parenthetical remarks as they grow.

7.1.2. Development of Voice

The fundamental frequency of the birth cry is as high as about 600 Hz. In infants the fundamental frequency is around 400 Hz and decreases till puberty. The fundamental frequency decreases significantly in boys but not so in girls at puberty. Fundamental frequency increases during senescence in males and decreases in females. The normal fundamental frequency in adult males is between 80 Hz to 180 Hz and in adult females it is between 180 Hz to 280 Hz. However, fundamental frequency may vary depending on culture, role model etc.

7.1.3. Development of Language

Language develops in gradual hierarchical steps from infancy to puberty. A child born has no language but communicates his/her basic needs through cry. Speech, i.e., vocal language develops naturally without any formal training. Majority of children exhibit several identifiable stages in speech and language development as the following.

Sl. No.	Stage	Age
1	Cooing	6 weeks
2	Babbling	6 months
3	Intonational patterns	8 months
4	1 – word utterances	1 year
5	2 – word utterances	18 months
6	Word inflections	2 years
7	Questions and negatives	2.6 years
8	Complex constructions	5 years
9	Matured speech	10 years

Language has several components viz. phonology, morphology, syntax, semantics, and pragmatics. Within each of the five components of language, development is seldom linear. At times, one aspect or a combination may be the major focus of development, as in the early stage when semantics and

28   S. R. Savithri

pragmatics appear to be the organizing features of child language. Later stage has numerous syntactic structures. This growth slows down in the school age years.

7.1.4. Speech and Language Development

Basically, the aspects discussed above may be identified as speech, language and communication milestones stage wise, as described below. It incorporates both expression and comprehension.

0-6 months
Expression
- Repeats the same sounds
- Frequently coos, gurgles, and makes pleasure sounds
- Uses different cry to express different needs
- Smiles when spoken to
- Uses phonemes /b/, /p/, and /m/ in babbling
- Uses sounds or gestures to indicate wants

Comprehension
- Recognizes voices
- Localizes sounds by turning head
- Listens to speech

7-12 months
Expression
- Babbles using long and short groups of sounds
- Uses a song like pattern when babbling
- Uses speech sounds rather than only crying to get attention
- Uses sound approximations
- Begins to change babbling to jargon
- Uses speech intentionally for the first time
- Uses nouns almost exclusively
- Has an expressive vocabulary of 1-3 words

Comprehension

- Understands no and not
- Responds to simple requests
- Understands and responds to own name
- Listens to and imitates sounds
- Recognizes words for common items
- Listens when spoke to
- Understands simple commands

13-18 months
Expression

- Uses adult like intonation patterns
- Uses echolalia and jargon
- Uses jargon to fill gaps in fluency
- Omits some initial consonants and almost all final consonants
- Produces mostly unintelligible speech
- Has an expressive vocabulary of 3 to 20 or more words
- Combines gestures and vocalization
- Makes requests for more of desired items

Comprehension

- Follows simple commands
- identifies 1 to 3 body parts

19-24 months
Expression

- Uses words more frequently than jargon
- Has an expressive vocabulary of 50 to 100 or more words
- Starts to combine nouns and verbs
- Begins to use pronouns
- Maintains unstable voice control
- Uses appropriate intonation for questions
- Is approximately 25-50% intelligible to strangers
- Answers, "What's that" questions

- Knows body parts
- Accurately names a few familiar objects

Comprehension
- Enjoys listening to stories
- Has a receptive vocabulary of 300 or more words

2-3 years

Expression
- Speech is 50-75% intelligible
- Verbalizes toilet needs
- Requests items by name
- Points to pictures in a book when named
- Identifies several body parts
- Asks 1- or 2-word questions
- Uses 3- or 4-word phrases
- Uses some prepositions, articles, present progressive verbs, regular plurals, contractions, and irregular past tense forms
- Uses words that are general in context
- Continues use of echolalia when difficulties in speech are encountered
- Has an expressive vocabulary of 50-250 or more words
- Exhibits multiple grammatical errors
- Frequently exhibits repetitions especially starters, I, and first syllables
- Speaks with a loud voice
- Increases range of pitch
- Uses vowels correctly
- Consistently uses initial consonants
- Frequently omits medial consonants
- Frequently omits or substitutes final consonants
- Uses approximately 27 phonemes
- Uses auxiliary is including the contracted form

Speech, Language and Communication

- Uses some regular past tense verbs, possessive morphemes, phonemes, pronouns, and imperatives

Comprehension

- Understands one and all
- Follows simple commands and answers simple questions
- Enjoys listening to short stories, songs, and rhymes
- Has a receptive vocabulary of 500 – 900 or more words
- Understands most things said to him or her

3-4 years

Expression

- Asks and answers simple questions
- Frequently asks questions and often demands detail in responses
- Produces simple verbal analogies
- Uses language to express emotions
- Uses 4 to 5-word sentences
- Repeats 6 to 13 syllable sentences accurately
- Identifies objects by name
- Manipulates adults and peers
- May continue to use echolalia
- Uses up to 6 words in a sentence
- Uses nouns and verbs most frequently
- Is conscious of past and future
- Has 800 to 1500 or more expressive vocabulary
- May repeat self often, exhibiting blocks, disturbed breathing, and facial grimaces during speech
- Increases speech rate
- Whispers
- Masters 50% of consonants and blends
- Speech is 80% intelligible
- Sentence grammar improves, although some errors still persist
- Approximately uses is, are, and am in sentences
- Tells two events in chronological order

- Engages in long conversations
- Uses some contractions, irregular plurals, future tense verbs, and conjunctions
- Consistently uses regular plurals, possessives, and simple past tense verbs

Comprehension
- Understands object functions
- Understands differences in meanings
- Follows 2- and 3-part commands
- Has a receptive vocabulary of 1,200 to 2000 or more

4-5 years
Expression
- Imitatively counts to 5
- Counts to by rote
- Answers questions about function
- Uses grammatically correct sentences
- Has an expressive vocabulary of 900 to 2000 or more words
- Uses sentences of 4 to 8 words
- Answers complex 2-part questions
- Asks for word definitions
- Speaks at a rate of approximately 80-180 words per minute
- Reduces total number of repetitions
- Enjoys rhymes, and nonsense syllables
- Produces consonants with 90% accuracy
- Significantly reduces number of persistent sound omissions and substitutions
- Frequently omits medial consonants
- Speech is usually intelligible to strangers
- Talks about experiences at school, at friend's house, etc.
- Uses some irregular plurals, possessive pronouns, future tense, reflexive pronouns, and comparative morphemes in sentences

Speech, Language and Communication 33

Comprehension
- Understands concept of numbers up to 3
- Continues understanding of spatial concepts
- Recognizes 1 to 3 colors
- Has a receptive vocabulary of 2800 or more words
- Listens to short, simple stories
- Pays attention to a story and answers simple questions about it

Following this, language develops and is complete by around 7 years of age.

8. PRE-REQUISITES AND FACTORS AFFECTING SPEECH-LANGUAGE DEVELOPMENT

The pre-requisites for speech and language development are an intact nervous system, respiratory system, laryngeal system, and resonatory system. Further, hearing, cognitive and motor development should be normal, and the child should get sufficient speech stimulation.

Following are some general factors affecting speech and language development. Some of these are to do with the child and some with the environment. Some of the factors within the child that affects speech and language development are global developmental delay, specific language impairment, poor motor co-ordination, medical conditions, hearing impairment, and lack of communication intent. *Global development delay* results in delay in developing motor skills which is especially essential for movements of all muscles including muscles required for speech production. It also results in delay in cognitive development the consequence of which will be mental retardation. With a delay in cognitive development all cognitive activities are delayed including speech and language. *Specific language impairment* refers to delay in language development which can't be attributed to global developmental delay, autism spectrum disorder, apraxia, brain damage or hearing loss. The causes are attributed to auditory temporal processing (Ceponiene, Cummings, Wulfeck, Ballantyne & Townsend, 2009; Tallal, 2004), specialized language learning system (Rice, Wexler, & Cleve, 1995; *van der* Lely, 2005), and memory (Lum, Gelgic, & Conti-Ramsden, 2010; Ullman & Pierpont, 2005). *Poor motor co-ordination of the speech muscles* may result from several medical conditions including cerebral palsy. Speech muscle coordination is essential for the movement of articulators to produce speech sounds. Incoordination results in improper movement of articulators effecting speech production. Several *medical conditions*, in general, retard the development including development of speech and language. These include dysarthria, tongue tie, paralysis, seizures, cleft palate etc. *Hearing loss*, especially sensory-neural hearing loss, is a cause of delayed speech and language development. The child is unable to hear others speak, in addition to lack of feedback of his speech resulting in delayed development of speech and language. *Emotional factors* such as behavioral problems, anxiety, pressure to perform etc. also results in delay in development of speech and language. *Short attention span* is also a factor affecting speech and language development. Memory is essential for a child to retain the phonemes/ words to communicate. With a short attention span, storage and hence retention of phonemes/ words is difficult. Further, *lack of communication intent,* as in autism spectrum disorders, may also be a factor affecting development of speech and language. Though all systems involving the development of speech and language are normal, the child may not develop normal speech and language owing of lack of interest in communication.

Environment factors include inadequate speech stimulation, frequent changes in the child's environment, exposure to several languages, family history of delayed speech and language, and inadequate opportunity for the child to speak. The child basically learns to speak by listening to others speak. Under circumstances of *inadequate speech stimulation*, in spite of all other things being normal, the child may not develop normal speech and language. Children usually have groups to communicate. Shifting of family very often results in *frequent shifting of environment*, and the child is unable to adjust to the new environment quickly; or the care taker may be changing too frequently. *Exposure to multiple languages* has not been proved to delay the development of speech and language. However, it may be a possible factor with the child mixing the codes of various languages. Often, the family members consider the child to be too young to reply and engage in conversation and talk for the child. OR a dominant sibling may be talking for the child. None of these provide *adequate opportunity for speech* and results in delay in the development of speech and language. *Family history of delayed speech and language* may also be a factor affecting development of speech and language. Apart from the above, multitude of economic factors influences the development of speech and language. Families in lower socio-economic status, families living under stress, unavailability of safe housing, not having the resources to provide food and nourishment, not having access to health care services, and not having enough financial security influence the development of speech and language. Factors such as parent education levels and parental attitudes toward education may lead to delay in language development in their children. In contrast, higher parental education levels and parental knowledge of school functions are important factors to encourage language and academic growth in bilingual children. Children of teenage mothers often have poor speech and language development. The home literary environment also influences receptive and expressive vocabulary growth during the later years of life.

9. CULTURAL AND LINGUISTIC ISSUES IN COMMUNICATION; BI/MULTILINGUAL ISSUES

India is a multilingual and multicultural country. Languages spoken in India belong to several language families. Indo-Aryan languages are spoken by 75% of Indians and the Dravidian languages spoken by 20% of Indians. The remaining 5% of languages belong to the Austro-Asiatic, Sino-Tibetan, Tai-Kadai, and a few other minor language families and isolates. According to Census of India of 2001, India has 122 major languages and 1599 other languages. India (780) has the world's second highest number of languages, after Papua New Guinea (839).

As per Article 343 of the Indian constitution the official language of the Union government is Hindi in Devanagari script. But it is superseded by English subsequently too as mentioned in section 3 of the same constitutional article that is put to effect by The Official Languages Act, 1963. The Government of India has awarded the distinction of *classical language* to Tamil, Sanskrit, Kannada, Telugu, Malayalam and Odia.

Language is a social-cultural-geographical phenomenon. There is an intricate relationship between language, culture and society. Child acquires and uses language in society. Therefore, it is essential to study the dialects, sociolects, idiolects, etc. of a language.

Hence, one has to keep in mind the geographical and cultural area in which this language is spoken, the society in which it is used, the speakers who use it, the listeners for whom it is used, and the purpose for which it is used, in addition to the linguistic components. Only then the study of a language can be complete and comprehensive. So, one must study language from the points of view of both form, and functions in culture. Socio-linguistics is the study of speech functions according to the speaker, the hearer, their relationship and contact, the context and the situation, the topic of discourse, the purpose of discourse, and the form of discourse. It studies the causes and consequences of linguistic behavior in human societies; it is concerned with the function of language, and studies language form without. Thus, there exist a unique bond between language and culture. For Saussure: "There is an absolute relation between language and culture."

Socio-linguistics is the study of linguistic realizations of socio-cultural meanings. The linguistic realizations may be both familiar and unfamiliar. The occurrence of everyday social interactions is relative to particular cultures, societies, social groups, speech communities, languages, dialects, varieties, styles. That is the reason that language variation forms a part of socio-linguistic study. Language can vary, not only from one individual to the next, but also from one sub-section of speech-community (family, village, town, and region) to another. People of different age, gender, social classes, occupations, or cultural groups in the same community may show variations in their speech. Therefore, language varies in geographical and social space. According to socio-linguists, a language is code. Each

Speech, Language and Communication 37

individual has some idiosyncratic linguistic features in his/ her use of language. These personal linguistic features are known as *Idiolect*. David crystal defines Idiolect as: "Idiolect refers to Linguistic system of an individual—one's personal dialect"

Human beings thinking, choice, and behavior vary according to need and situation. Along with the behavior adaptation, they adapt their language also, which forms language variety called '*Register*'. Register is social variation and dialect is geographical variation. Crystal asserts that "Register is a variety of language defined according to its use in a social situation" Unlike register, *Dialect* is a variety of language which has its peculiar vocabulary, grammar, and pronunciation.

Other varieties of language that develop due to the cultural pressure are *Pidgin and Creole*. Pidgin refers to an 'odd mixture' of two languages. It is not a divergent variety of 'a language' but a combination of two or more languages. Languages are mixed up oddly and everything from morphemes to sentence structure reduces and combines strangely. Most of the present pidgins have developed in European colonies. A few examples are Hawaii Creole English and Tok Pisin, Bislama. After a certain period of time Pidgin is used as native language which is termed Creoles. While Pidgin has no native speakers, Creole has. Creole develops its new structures and vocabulary. Crystal defines pidgin as "A language with a markedly reduced grammatical structure, lexicon, and stylistic range, formed by two mutually unintelligible speech communities."

Therefore, language and culture are complementary to each other. Language cannot exist without society. Language varieties are due to cultural and social needs. Further, language of an individual varies from occasion to occasion. There are different levels of formalities with in a language and their use depends of speaker's purpose, mode and audience. It also varies due to socio-economic position of individual or group. This variation of language with social difference, affirms that language is a social and cultural phenomenon and is coupled with social and cultural traditions. The study of Esperanto also revealed this fact that language and culture are inseparable.

Several terms have been used to designate culturally and linguistically diverse (CLD) population. Nieto (2004) defines culture as "values, traditions, social and political relationship, and a world created, shared, and transformed by a group of people bound together by a common history, geographic location and language, social class, religion or other shared identity." As one can observe "culture" includes aspects of a group to identity that has some observable pattern such as traditions and social relationships. In addition, language is embedded in the definition. Two speakers of the same language may communicate verbally and nonverbally, but in a different way depending on age, education, gender, social class etc. Verbal communication may be easier to describe as it has components such as words, sentences etc. However, nonverbal communication is difficult to interpret as it depends on the backgrounds and cultures of the persons who interact with each other.

The concept of culture keeps evolving with time. For example, Kannada speakers when speaking with Speaker with Hindi or English as their mother tongue tends to use borrowed words from these languages as it would be essential. And therefore, while the older generations tend to retain the culture in the original form, the younger generation may not.

In addition to culture and language, race and ethnicity are terms that are frequently used interchangeably to mark distinctions between several groups. Race is primarily to do with physical characteristics such as skin color and facial features, and ethnicity adds on to the idea of customs, values, ancestry, tradition, religion, and history (Trumbull & Farr, 2005).

A Speech-Language Pathologist, in India, with a background of one/two languages finds it difficult to assess and rehabilitate persons with speech/ language disorders speaking a different language and as such s/he may require assistance. In the process of assessing the speech, language and communication skills of an individual, his/her language, race, ethnicity, age, gender, experience, contact with individuals speaking other languages, education, economic opportunities, personality, and motivation should also be considered. The following are the prominent languages of India and is taken from https://en.wikipedia.org/wiki/Languages_of_India.

Speech, Language and Communication 39

9.1. Bengali

It is native to the Bengal region, comprising the nation of Bangladesh and the states of West Bengal, Tripura and Barak Valley region of Assam. Bengali is the fifth most spoken language in the world. After partition of India (1947), refugees from East Pakistan were settled in Tripura, and Jharkhand and the union territory of Andaman and Nicobar Islands. There are also a large number of Bengali-speaking people in Maharashtra and Gujarat where they work as artisans in jewellery industries. Bengali developed from Abahatta, a derivative of Apabhramsha, itself derived from Magadhi Prakrit. The modern Bengali vocabulary contains the vocabulary base from Magadhi Prakrit and Pali, also borrowings & reborrowing's from Sanskrit and other major borrowings from Persian, Arabic, Austro-Asiatic languages and other languages in contact with. Like most Indian languages, Bengali has a number of dialects. Interestingly it exhibits diglossia, with the literary and standard form differing greatly from the colloquial speech of the regions that identify with the language. Bengali language has developed a rich cultural base spanning art, music, literature and religion. There have been many movements in defence of this language and in 1999 UNESCO declared 21 Feb as the International Mother Language Day in commemoration of the Bengali Language Movement in 1952.

9.2. Telugu

Telugu is the most widely spoken Dravidian language in India. Telugu is an official language in Andhra Pradesh, Telangana and the union territory of Puducherry, making it one of the few languages (along with Hindi, Bengali, and Urdu) with official status in more than one state. It is also spoken by significant minorities in the Andaman and Nicobar Islands, Chhattisgarh, Karnataka, Maharashtra, Odisha, Tamil Nadu, and by the Sri Lankan Gypsy people. It is one of six languages with classical status in India. Telugu ranks third by the number of native speakers in India (74 million in

40   *S. R. Savithri*

the 2001 Census), fifteenth in the *Ethnologue* list of most-spoken languages worldwide and is the most widely spoken Dravidian language.

9.3. Marathi

Marathi is an Indo-Aryan language. It is the official language and co-official language in Maharashtra and Goa states of Western India respectively, and is one of the official languages of India. There were 71 million speakers in 2001 and 73 million speakers in 2007, ranking 19th in the list of most spoken languages. Marathi has the fourth largest number of native speakers in India. Marathi has some of the oldest literature of all modern Indo-Aryan languages, dating from about 1200 AD (Mukundraj's *Vivek Sindhu* from the close of the 12th century). The major dialects of Marathi are Standard Marathi and the Varhadi dialect. There are other related languages such as Khandeshi, Dangi, Vadvali and Samavedi. Malvani Konkani is heavily influenced by Marathi varieties. Marathi is one of several languages that descend from Maharashtri Prakrit. Further change led to the Apabhraṃśa languages like Old Marathi.

Marathi is the official language of Maharashtra and co-official language in the union territories of Daman and Diu and Dadra and Nagar Haveli. In Goa, Konkani is the sole official language; however, Marathi may also be used for all official purposes.

Over a period of many centuries the Marathi language and people came into contact with many other languages and dialects. The primary influence of Prakrit, Maharashtri, Dravidian languages, Apabhraṃśa and Sanskrit is understandable. At least 50% of the words in Marathi are either taken or derived from Sanskrit. Many scholars claim that Sanskrit has derived many words from Marathi. Marathi has also shared directions, vocabulary and grammar with languages such as Indian Dravidian languages, and foreign languages such as Persian, Arabic, English and a little from Portuguese.

9.4. Tamil

Tamil is a Dravidian language predominantly spoken in Tamil Nadu, Puducherry and many parts of Sri Lanka. It is also spoken by large minorities in the Andaman and Nicobar Islands, Kerala, Karnataka, Andhra Pradesh, Malaysia, Singapore, Mauritius and throughout the world. Tamil ranks fourth by the number of native speakers in India (72 million in the 2001 Census) and ranks 20th in the list of most spoken languages. It is one of the 22 scheduled languages of India and was the first Indian language to be declared a classical language by the Government of India in 2004. Tamil is one of the longest surviving classical languages in the world. It has been described as "the only language of contemporary India which is recognizably continuous with a classical past." The two earliest manuscripts from India, acknowledged and registered by UNESCO Memory of the World register in 1997 and 2005, are in Tamil. Tamil is an official language of Tamil Nadu, Puducherry, Andaman and Nicobar Islands, Sri Lanka and Singapore. It is also recognized as minority language in Canada, Malaysia, Mauritius and South Africa.

9.5. Urdu

After independence, Modern Standard Urdu, the Persianized register of Hindustani became the national language of Pakistan. During British colonial times, knowledge of Hindustani or Urdu was a must for officials. Hindustani was made the second language of British Indian Empire after English and considered as the language of administration. The British introduced the use of Roman script for Hindustani as well as other languages. Urdu had 70 million speakers in India (as per the Census of 2001), and, along with Hindi, is one of the 22 officially recognized regional languages of India and also an official language in the Indian states of Jammu and Kashmir, Delhi, Uttar Pradesh, Bihar and Telangana that have significant Muslim populations.

42

9.6. Gujarati

Gujarati is an Indo-Aryan language. It is native to the West Indian region of Gujarat. Gujarati is part of the greater Indo-European language family. Gujarati is descended from Old Gujarati (c. 1100 – 1500 CE), the same source as that of Rajasthani. Gujarati is the chief language in the Indian state of Gujarat. It is also an official language in the union territories of Daman and Diu and Dadra and Nagar Haveli. According to the Central Intelligence Agency (CIA), 4.5% of population of India (1.21 billion according to 2011 census) speaks Gujarati. This amounts to 54.6 million speakers in India.

9.7. Kannada

Kannada language is a Dravidian language which branched off from Kannada-Tamil sub group around 500 B.C.E according to the Dravidian scholar Zvelebil. According to the Dravidian scholars Steever and Krishnamurthy, the study of Kannada language is usually divided into three linguistic phases: Old (450–1200 CE), Middle (1200–1700 CE) and Modern (1700–present). The earliest written records are from the 5th century, and the earliest available literature in rich manuscript (*Kavira:jama:rga*) is from c. 850. Kannada language has the second oldest written tradition of all vernacular languages of India. Current estimates of the total number of epigraph present in Karnataka range from 25,000 by the scholar Sheldon Pollock to over 30,000 by the Sahitya Akademi, making Karnataka state "one of the most densely inscribed pieces of real estate in the world." According to Garg and Shipely, more than a thousand notable writers have contributed to the wealth of the language.

9.8. Malayalam

Malayalam has official language status in the state of Kerala and in the union territories of Lakshadweep and Puducherry. It belongs to the

Speech, Language and Communication 43

Dravidian family of languages and is spoken by some 38 million people. Malayalam is also spoken in the neighboring states of Tamil Nadu and Karnataka; with some speakers in the Nilgiris, Kanyakumari and Coimbatore districts of Tamil Nadu, and the Dakshina Kannada and the Kodagu district of Karnataka. Malayalam originated from Middle Tamil (Sen-Tamil) in the 7th century. As Malayalam began to freely borrow words as well as the rules of grammar from Sanskrit, the Grantha alphabet was adopted for writing and came to be known as *Arya Eluttu*. This developed into the modern Malayalam script.

9.9. Odia

Odia (formerly spelled *Oriya*) is the only Indian classical language from Indo-Aryan group. Odia is primarily spoken in the Indian state of Odisha and has over 40 million speakers. It was declared as a classical language of India in 2014. Native speakers comprise 80% of the population in Odisha. Odia is thought to have originated from Magadhi Prakrit similar to Ardha Magadhi, a language spoken in eastern India over 1,500 years ago. The history of Odia language can be divided to Old Odia (7th century–1200), Early Middle Odia (1200–1400), Middle Odia (1400–1700), Late Middle Odia (1700–1850) and Modern Odia (1850 till present day). The National Manuscripts Mission of India has found around 213,000 unearthed and preserved manuscripts written in Odia.

9.10. Punjabi

Punjabi, written in the Gurmukhi script in India, is one of the prominent languages of India with about 32 million speakers. In Pakistan it is spoken by over 80 million people and is written in the Shahmukhi alphabet. It is mainly spoken in Punjab but also in neighboring areas. It is an official language of Delhi.

9.11. Assamese

Asamiya or Assamese language is most popular in the state of Assam and Brahmaputra Valley. It's an Eastern Indo-Aryan language having more than 10 million speakers as per world estimates by Encarta.

9.12. Maithili

Maithili is an Indo-Aryan language spoken in the Mithila region which is today mainly situated in northern and eastern Bihar of India and a few districts of the Nepal Terai. The 2001 estimated percentage of Indians speaking this language was 1.18%. It is the second most prevalent language spoken in Nepal.

Less commonly, it was written with a Maithili variant of Kaithi, a script used to transcribe other neighboring languages such as Bhojpuri, Magahi, and Awadhi.

In 2002, Maithili was included in the Eighth Schedule of the Indian Constitution as a recognized regional language of India, which allows it to be used in education, government, and other official contexts.

The 2001 census identified the following native languages having more than one million speakers. Most of them are dialects/variants grouped under Hindi.

Apart from the languages spoken in India, there are several other languages of the world which can be grouped in to different language families. *Language family* refers to a group of languages related by a descent from a common *ancestral language* or *parental language*, called the *proto-language* of that family. Linguists describe the *daughter languages* within a language family as being *genetically related.*

A *living language* is one that is used by a group of people as the primary form of communication. There are several dead and extinct languages, and some languages that are still insufficiently studied to be classified, or are even unknown outside their respective speech communities.

Speech, Language and Communication 45

Languages	No. of native speakers
Bhojpuri	33,099,497
Rajasthani	18,355,613
Magadhi/Magahi	13,978,565
Chhattisgarhi	13,260,186
Haryanvi	7,997,192
Marwari	7,936,183
Malvi	5,565,167
Mewari	5,091,697
Khorth / Khotta	4,725,927
Bundeli	3,072,147
Bagheli	2,865,011
Pahari	2,832,825
Laman /Lambadi	2,707,562
Awadhi	2,529,308
Harauti	2,462,867
Garhwali	2,267,314
Nimadi	2,148,146
Sadan /Sadri	2,044,776
Kumauni	2,003,783
Dhundhari	1,871,130
Tulu	1,722,768
Surgujia	1,458,533
Bagri Rajasthani	1,434,123
Banjari	1,259,821
Nagpuria (Varhadi)	1,242,586
Surajpuri	1,217,019
Sylheti	3,612,653
Kangri	1,122,843

Genealogically related languages show shared preservations. Features of the proto-language cannot be explained by chance or borrowing.

Language families can be divided into smaller phylogenetic units which are referred to as *branches* of the family as the history of a language family is often represented as a tree diagram.

Following are the families containing at least 1% of the 7,472 known languages in the world by *Ethnologue* 18 (https://en.wikipedia.org/wiki/List_of_language_families):

1) Niger–Congo (1,538 languages) (20.6%)
2) Austronesian (1,257 languages) (16.8%)

3) Trans–New Guinea (480 languages) (6.4%)
4) Sino-Tibetan (457 languages) (6.1%)
5) Indo-European (444 languages) (5.9%)
6) Australian (378 languages) (5.1%)
7) Afro-Asiatic (375 languages) (5.0%)
8) Nilo-Saharan (205 languages) (2.7%)
9) Oto-Manguean (177 languages) (2.4%)
10) Austro-Asiatic (169 languages) (2.3%)
11) Volta–Congo (108 languages) (1.5%)
12) Tai–Kadai (95 languages) (1.3%)
13) Dravidian (85 languages) (1.1%)
14) Tupian (76 languages) (1.0%)

CONCLUSION

The chapter covered definitions of speech, language, communication, and their components. Components of speech included voice and its components, oral structure, place and manner of articulation under articulation, fluency, and prosody. Components of language included phonology, syntax, semantics, and pragmatics. Components of communication included (a) context, (b) sender/encoder/ source, (c) message, (d) medium/ channel, (e) receiver/decoder, (f) effect, and (g) feedback. Distinctions, similarities and functions of communication, speech and language were discussed. The chapter also included how speech is an overlaid function along with speech chain from speaker to listener. Normal development of speech sounds, development of fluency, development of voice, and development of language were included. Further, pre-requisites and factors affecting speech-language development, and cultural and linguistic issues in communication; bi/multilingual issues were covered. Under cultural and linguistic issues, language families and a note about Indian languages were also covered.

Speech, Language and Communication 47

REFERENCES

Ceponiene, R., Cummings, A., Wulfeck, B., Ballantyne, A., and Townsend, J. 2009. "Spectral vs. temporal auditory processing in specific language impairment: A developmental ERP study." *Brain & Language*. 110 (3): 107–20. PMC 2731814. PMID 19457549. doi:10.1016/j.bandl. 2009.04.003.

Crystal, D. 2007. *The Fight for English: How Language Pundits Ate, Shot, and Left*, Oxford: Oxford University Press.

Encyclopædia Britannica Online. Retrieved from https://www.britannica. com/. Accessed May 10.

Hindi languages. *Encyclopædia Britannica Online*. Retrieved from https://www.soas.ac.uk/southasia/languages/hindi/Accessed May 10.

https://en.wikipedia.org/wiki/Languages_of_India. Accessed May 10.

https://en.wikipedia.org/wiki/List_of_language_families. Accessed May 10.

Justice, L. M. 2010. *Communication Sciences and Disorders: A Contemporary Perspective* (2nd Ed.). Boston: Allyn & Bacon.

Khara, L. P. T. and Laura M. J. 2011. *Language Development from Theory to Practice (Communication Sciences and Disorders)* (2nd Ed.), UK: Pearson publications.

Lum, J. A., Gelgic, C., and Conti-Ramsden, G. 2010. "Procedural and declarative memory in children with and without specific language impairment." *Int J Lang Commun Disord*. 45(1):96-107. PMC 2826154 . PMID 19900077. doi:10.3109/13682820902752285.

Leonard, L. B. 1998. *Children with specific language impairment*. Cambridge, MA: MIT Press.

Nieto, S. 2004. *Affirming diversity. The socio-political context of multicultural education* (4th Ed.). Boston: Pearson.

Official Language Act | Government of India, Ministry of Electronics and Information Technology. Retrieved from meity.gov.in. Accessed May 10.

Rice, M. L., Wexler, K., and Cleave, P. L. 1995. "Specific language impairment as a period of extended optional infinitive." *J Speech Hear*

48   S. R. Savithri

Res. 38 (4): 850–63. PMID 7474978. doi:10.1044/jshr.3804.850. Tallal, 2004.

Shames, G. H., Wiig, E. H., and Secord. W. A. 1998. *Human Communication Disorders.* Boston: Allyn and Bacon.

Starkweather, C. W. 1987. *Fluency and stuttering.* Englewood Cliffs, New Jersey: Prentice-Hall.

Tallal. P. 2004. "Improving language and literacy is a matter of time." *Nat. Rev. Neurosci. 5 (9): 721–8.* PMID 15322530. doi:10.1038/nrn1499.

Trumbull, E., & Farr, B. 2005. *Language and learning. What teachers used to know.* Norwood, MA: Christopher Gordon.

Turnbull, K. L., & Justice, L. M. 2008. *Language Development from Theory to Practice.* New Jersey: Pearson Education, Inc.

Ullman, M. T., & Pierpont, E. I. 2005. "Specific language impairment is not specific to language: the procedural deficit hypothesis." *Cortex.* 41 (3): 399–433. PMID 15871604. doi:10.1016/s0010-9452(08)70276-4.

van der Lely, H. K. 2005. "Domain-specific cognitive systems: insight from Grammatical-SLI." *Trends Cogn. Sci. (Regul. Ed.).* 9 (2): 53–9. PMID 15668097. doi:10.1016/j.tics.2004.12.002.

Chapter 2

BASES OF SPEECH AND LANGUAGE

INTRODUCTION

Sound is a vibration that transmits as audible mechanical wave of pressure and displacement, through a medium such as air or water. It is essential to know about the generation and properties of sound as speech also is considered as a sound generated by the source AIR. Sound can be a simple or a complex wave; but speech is always a complex wave. Speech is a sound produced by the air passing through the lungs and modified by the vibrating vocal folds, and articulators. Several systems – the nervous system, the respiratory system, the laryngeal system, and resonatory / articulatory system – contribute and should work typically to produce normal speech. Abnormalities in any of these systems will cause abnormal speech. Speech and language are considered to be learnt by some authors and as innate by some. Further to the various systems, it is also important that the child receives sufficient speech stimulation from the society/ caretakers/ parents/ siblings. It is also known that genetic abnormalities of speech & language in parents transmit to children who in turn might inherit these defects. Therefore, various systems in the human body, the society, and the genetics apart from others form the bases of speech.

1. Overview of Speech Production – Speech Sub-Systems

1.1. Speech Production – Speech Sub-Systems

Several systems in the human body help in speech production. These include (a) nervous system, (b) respiratory system, (c) phonatory system, and (d) articulatory or resonatory system.

1.2. Nervous System

The nervous system is the part of a human being that coordinates its actions by transmitting signals to and from different parts of its body. It consists of two main parts, the central nervous system (CNS) and the peripheral nervous system (PNS). The CNS consists of the brain and spinal cord.

The PNS consists of nerves, which are enclosed bundles of axons or long fibers. These nerves connect the CNS to parts of the body. There are two types of nerves, motor or efferent and sensory or afferent. Nerves that transmit signals from the brain to the other parts of the body are called motor nerves (for example movement of fingers) and the nerves that transmit information from the body to the CNS are called sensory nerves (for example sensation of pain). Spinal nerves serve both motor and sensory functions and are termed mixed nerves.

The PNS has three separate subsystems, the somatic, autonomic, and enteric nervous systems. Somatic nerves are responsible for voluntary movement. Autonomic nervous system has sympathetic and parasympathetic nervous systems. The sympathetic nervous system is activated in cases of emergencies to gather energy and the parasympathetic nervous system is activated when the organism is in a relaxed state. The enteric nervous system controls the gastrointestinal system. Functions of both autonomic and enteric nervous systems are involuntary in nature.

Bases of Speech and Language 51

Cranial nerves are those exiting from the cranium and spinal nerves are those exiting from the spinal cord.

There are 12 pairs of cranial nerves which innervate different organs in the head and neck region (except Vagus nerve) and are important in speech production. The names of these nerves follow their structure or function. Table 3 shows the name, origin, innervation, and function.

Table 3. Cranial nerves with their functions

Sl. No.	Name of the cranial nerve	Function
1)	Olfactory nerve	Sensory - smell
2)	Optic Nerve	Sensory - visual
3)	Oculomotor nerve	Motor - visual
4)	Trochlear nerve	Motor - visual
5)	Trigeminal nerve	Mixed – Jaw, lips, face, tongue
6)	Abducens nerve	Motor - visual
7)	Facial nerve	Mixed - tongue, soft palate, face, lips, and the stapedius muscle of the middle ear
8)	Vestibulocochlear nerve	Sensory – vestibule, cochlea
9)	Glossopharyngeal nerve	Mixed – tongue, pharynx
10)	Vagus nerve	Mixed - larynx, pharynx, soft palate, thoracic and abdominal viscera
11)	Accessory nerve	Motor – neck, shoulder
12)	Hypoglossal nerve	Motor - tongue

The brain embedded inside the head or skull, has two hemispheres – the left and the right. Each hemisphere has 4 parts or lobes – (a) frontal lobe which is situated in front, (b) temporal lobe, just behind / above the external ears, (c) occipital lobe, at the back side, and (d) parietal lobe, in the center. Some regions in these lobes facilitate in speech production. When there is a desire to speak, Wernicke's area (41, 42), located in the parietal lobe, chooses the words to be spoken and prepares the word order and sends the message to speech motor areas. These include Broca's area (44) and area number 4 in the frontal lobe. These areas convert the message in to motor actions or they generate and send commands to other systems of speech production through nerves. Therefore, the nervous system controls the speech production and can be compared to a commander in an army.

Without the orders by the nervous system, other speech systems can't work. Figure 14 shows the speech areas in the cerebral hemisphere.

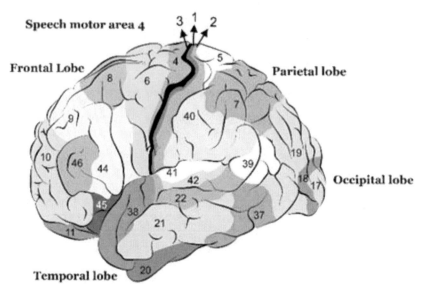

Source: https://www.slideshare.net/jeffarian/general-appearance-of-the-cerebral-hemispheres.

Figure 14. Speech areas of cerebral hemisphere.

The nervous system issues command to respiratory, laryngeal, and articulatory or resonatory systems.

1.3. Respiratory System

The respiratory system has two lungs at one end and the nostrils at the other end. The two lungs join together to form a tube called trachea. The trachea runs from lungs to throat. From there it enters the larynx and divides into mouth (oral tract) and nose (nasal tract). Figure 1 shows the respiratory system.

Bases of Speech and Language

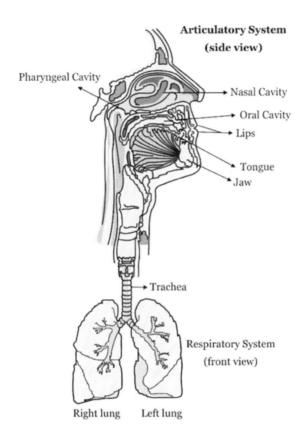

Figure 1. Respiratory, and articulatory system (lateral view). (Same figure as shown in Chapter 1).

The function of the respiratory system is respiration, which is the process of breathing for of gas exchange. It has two phases- inspiration and expiration. Air is breathed in during inspiration. Air enters the nose during inspiration and on reaching the lungs Oxygen is separated from air. Carbon Dioxide (CO_2) is breathed out during expiration. Air is pushed out of the lungs during expiration. Respiratory system acts like a pump, pumping the air in during inspiration and pumping the air out during expiration. Lungs expand during inspiration and contract during expiration. We inspire about 60 times per second. The lungs can be compared to a rubber band or a harmonium. The expiratory air is the source of speech production and therefore, the respiratory system supplies energy for speech. In quiet respiration, the air is breathed in and out through the nose. But, in speech production, expiration can be through mouth or nose. In quiet breathing, inspiration and expiration share 50% each. But inspiration is shorter, and expiration is longer for speech purposes. Pressure of air required to produce speech is about 5-8 cm of H_2O.

1.4. Laryngeal System

The laryngeal system consists of the larynx or the voice box, situated in between the trachea and the oral tract. It is made up of a bone, cartilages and muscles and is suspended in the neck. The most important part of the larynx is a pair of vocal folds. Figure 15 shows the larynx.

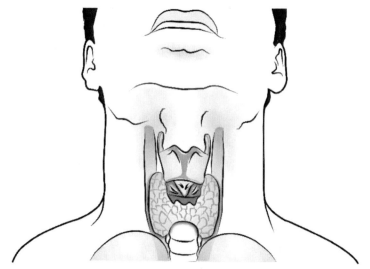

Source: https://www.google.com/search?q=larynx+in+adult+male&oq=larynx+in+adult+male&aqs=chrome.69i57.8719j1j4&sourceid=chrome&ie=UTF-8.

Figure 15. Larynx in an adult male.

The basic function of the vocal folds is to protect the lungs from foreign bodies. The vocal folds are like strings of a Veena. They vibrate when the air passes through them or open and close. The expiratory air is a stream of air and is equivalent to noise. When the vocal folds close, the air is stopped and when it is open the air is let out. Figure 16 illustrates the function of vocal folds.

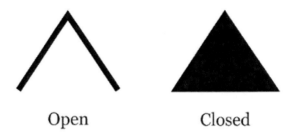

Figure 16. Illustration of the function of vocal folds.

During the vibration of the vocal folds, the stream of air or noise is modified into puffs of air or voice. This can be equated to a door opening and closing or clapping of hands. The length of the vocal folds is about 10-17 mm. The length changes with age and gender, being short in children and long in adults. They can vibrate anywhere between 80 times per second to 800 times per second. These small vocal folds produce amazing tones. One can't even imagine closing and opening a door 300 times per second mechanically and perhaps require a machine to do this. But the vocal folds can do this. We talk for hours without realizing the work of the miniature vocal folds. Keep your vocal folds healthy to have a clear and normal voice.

1.5. Resonatory/Articulatory System

The resonatory system includes (a) pharynx, the space above larynx, (b) mouth or the oral cavity, and (c) nose or the nasal cavity. The oral tract is separated from the nasal tract by the velopharyngeal port. When it is open, the expiratory air passes through the nasal tract, and during closure, the expiratory air passes through the oral tract. Figure 17 shows the resonatory system.

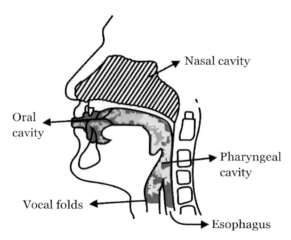

Source: https://en.wikipedia.org/wiki/Vocal_resonation.

Figure 17. The resonatory system.

The oral tract is like a box and you can consider the tongue to be the base of the box; palate to be the roof, teeth and lips to be the front parts. Though the primary function of all these organs in the oral tract is mastication, it also helps in speech production. The oral tract acts like a filter and can be compared to a sieve, which is the most common filter one comes across. Any filter retains some particles on the surface and passes the remaining as illustrated in Figure 18.

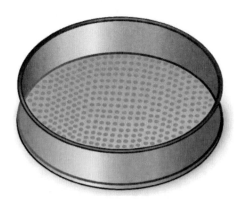

Source: https://en.wikipedia.org/wiki/Sieve.

Figure 18. A sieve.

Bases of Speech and Language

The vocal tract is about 17 cm in length and the articulators can be moved horizontally and vertically in the oral tract. Considering the vocal tract to be tube, it acts like a resonator. When the vocal tract is at rest, that is, when there is no movement of articulators in the tract, it resonates at 500 Hz, 1500 Hz, 2500 Hz etc. Consider saying /g/ sound several times. The back of the tongue touches the palate resulting in change in the shape and size of the vocal tract. The vocal tract is roughly divided in to two parts by virtue of closure of the tract in the velar region. At rest the vocal tract has some resonance frequencies. The expiratory air modified by the vibration of the vocal folds has energy at fundamental and several frequencies in it. It is further modified by the shape and size of the vocal tract which results in changes in resonance frequency. Energy in some frequencies is absorbed by the vocal tract and several of the frequencies are passed through the tract. Thus, the air coming out of the lips, speech, is source + filter function. In the production of /d/, the vocal tract is roughly divided in to two parts. Never the less, the shape and size of the vocal tract in the production of /d/ is different from that in the production of /g/ or these two are different filters. This filter also absorbs energy at some frequencies and passes energy at some frequencies. But it is not similar to /g/. Thus speech, the air, radiating from lips is different from /g/ because the filter is different. Figure 19 illustrates the filters created in the oral tract in producing /g/ and /d/.

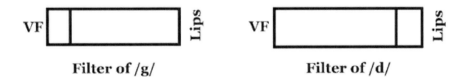

Figure 19. Illustration of the filters in the production of /g/ and /d/.

Therefore, the oral tract creates different filters by placing the tongue in different places, because of which the resonance frequencies change, and hence various speech sounds are produced.

58 *S. R. Savithri*

2. SPEECH MECHANISM AS A SOUND GENERATOR, VOCAL TRACT, PERIODIC AND APERIODIC SOUNDS

2.1. Sound

For any physical work some supply of energy is required. This physical work consists of converting the energy from one form to another. Sound generation is a physical work and hence it requires supply of energy.

In physics, "*sound* is a vibration that propagates as a typically audible mechanical wave of pressure and displacement, through a medium such as air or water. In physiology and psychology, sound is the *reception* of such waves and their *perception* by the brain" (*Fundamentals of Telephone Communication Systems*. Western Electric Company. 1969. p. 2.1). Sound is defined by ANSI/ASA S1.1-2013 as "(a) Oscillation in pressure, stress, particle displacement, particle velocity, etc., propagated in a medium with internal forces (e.g., elastic or viscous), or the superposition of such propagated oscillation. (b) Auditory sensation evoked by the oscillation described in (a)" (ANSI S1.1-1994. American National Standard: Acoustic Terminology. Sec 3.03).

2.2. Generation of Sound Waves

We shall start with a simple example of the sound generated by a tuning fork. Hold the tuning fork by the foot in your hand. It does not produce sound because there is no energy supplied and the tuning fork is at rest. Now strike the tuning fork on the knee or on a table. This will start the movement of the fork and set it on vibration. The energy that you supplied was stored in the metal and is being used up as to and fro movements of the left and right prongs. Figure 20 shows the tuning fork. See the movement of right prong of the tuning fork in Figure 21. Before it is struck the prong is in position A or the rest position. Once hit it moves to the left to position B. The distance from A to B will depend on how hard the prong is struck. The greater the force applied, the farther the prong will move. Now the prong is displaced from its rest position. In common with everything in nature, it will immediately try to get back to the rest position i.e., A. In the course of this movement it gathers momentum. As a result, it is unable to stop at position A and further moves to position C. As it has not assumed the resting position yet, it tries to move towards the rest position i.e., A. It overshoots and moves to position B and the movement continues until the energy is spent. We can assume that the distance between A to B is equal to the distance from A to C. The same movement happens in the left prong also. The movement of the prong from position A to A (A to B to A to C to A) makes one cycle of movement which is repeated several times. The distance from A to B or from A to C can be measured. Assume that a light weight pencil is stuck to the prong and the pencil is moving on a paper. When the tuning fork is at rest a straight line is drawn. When it is moving you will get a graph as shown in Figure 20 and the graph along with tuning fork is shown in Figure 23.

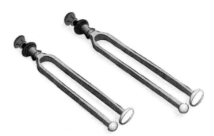

Source: https://www.google.com/search?q=tuning+forks&tbm=isch&source=univ&hl=en-IN&authuser=0&sa=X&sqi=2&ved=2ahUKEwi_r_HO5dHiAhXM7Z4KHc2NCKcQsAR6BAgAEAE&biw=1440&bih=735.

Figure 20. Tuning fork.

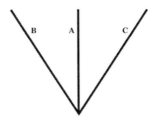

Figure 21. Motion of right prong of the tuning fork.

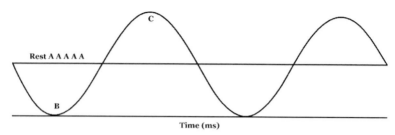

Source: http://www.arborsci.com/cool/top-10-demonstrations-with-tuning-forks.

Figure 22. Curve tracing motion of tuning fork prong.

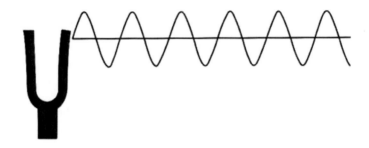

Figure 23. Tuning fork along with curve tracing motion.

Watch *http://www.arborsci.com/cool/top-10-demonstrations-with-tuning-forks* for demonstration of tuning forks. Tuning forks might have different frequencies of vibration. Figure 24 shows waves generated by two vibrating tuning forks.

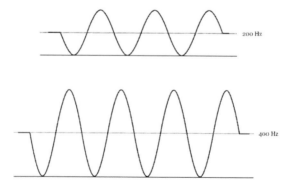

Figure 24. Waves of frequencies 200 Hz, and 400 Hz.

2.3. Cycle, Displacement, Period, Frequency, Amplitude

One *cycle* of movement of the tuning fork is the sequence A-B-A-C-A. In Figure 22, X axis represents time, and the instance at which the vibration begins is recorded as time 0. The distance from A to B or A C is termed *displacement*. Let us assume that the time taken from A-B-A is 2.5 ms and that taken from A-C-A is 2.5 ms. The total time taken to complete one cycle is 5 ms. Each cycle takes exactly the same time i.e., 5 ms. Owing to this regularity, 5 ms in this instance, the motion is said to be *periodic*. The *period* of vibration in this example is 5 ms. Frequency refers to the number of cycles per second. In this instance the tuning fork is taking 5 ms to complete one cycle and therefore it will complete 200 cycles per second (1000ms / 5 ms = 200). Hence the frequency of vibration is 200 cycles per second or 200 Hz (after the German Physicist, Heinrich Hertz). *Frequency* means the number of complete cycles per second. In every cycle of movement, the tuning fork is moving first to one side and then to the other of the position of rest. The measure of the displacement from position A to position B, or from position A to position C is referred to as the *amplitude* of vibration. If we hit the tuning fork hard, we hear a loud sound and when it is tapped, we hear a soft sound. So, the amplitude of the sound is linked with the sensation of loudness with louder sounds having higher amplitude. You can also observe that the sound generated by the tuning fork gradually fades and dies; the amplitude is decreasing until the prong of the fork comes to rest and there is no displacement from position A. This means that the distance between A and B or A and C are not equal from cycle to cycle; however, the changes takes place so slowly that the decrease in amplitude is not measurable. Figure 25 shows waveforms with different amplitudes.

Pitch is the perceptual correlate of frequency and loudness is the perceptual correlate of amplitude. We have understood and determined the frequency and amplitude of the simplest kind of sound. In order to understand the physical attributes of complex sound we need to consider a number of other factors that enter in to the vibratory motion.

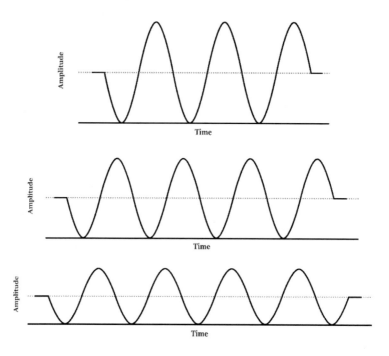

Figure 25. Waveforms with different amplitudes.

2.4. Simple Harmonic Motion, Sine Wave, Complex Wave

In case you hold the tuning fork by its stem with the prongs pointing to the ground and strike one of the prongs, the fork will begin to vibrate, and the motion of the prong resembles that of a pendulum as in Figure 26. A mark the position of rest and B and C mark the displacement.

As learnt earlier, we have to supply energy for the pendulum to vibrate. However, instead of striking the pendulum, the bob is drawn to one side from the rest position to position B. The bob will travel back to the rest position A, overshoot and travel to position B and will perform repeatedly the same cycle of motion. The swinging of the pendulum will be perfectly regular, that is each cycle of movement will take the same time which will determine the frequency of the oscillation. The frequency of the oscillations would be much lower than that of a tuning fork and may be 1 cycle per

Bases of Speech and Language 63

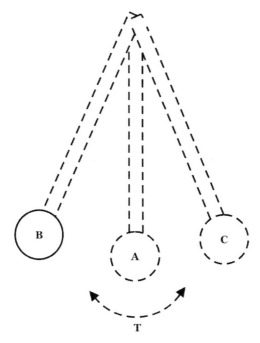

Source: http://www.pbs.org/opb/circus/classroom/circus-physics/pendulum-motion/.

Figure 26. Motion of a pendulum.

second. We do not hear a sound when a pendulum is swinging because the frequency of vibration is below the range required to produce the sensation of sound in the human ears. Consider attaching a light stylus to the bob of the pendulum and record the swings. We should obtain a similar graph as in Figure 22, except for the time scale. One cycle of the tuning fork vibration took 5 ms in the example above; one cycle of the pendulum vibration might take 1 second. The movement of the pendulum is better visible as it moves slowly. The movement performed by both the prong of the tuning fork and the pendulum is termed *simple harmonic motion*. Till now we understood about distance and the duration travelled by the prong or the bob. This motion has other properties also which may be considered. For example, we can consider how fast the bob is travelling at a given moment. The bob is swinging first to the left (position B) and then to the right (position C). So, there are two movements in each cycle when it reverses the direction. At this moment the bob must be stationary or no speed at all. When it travels back towards position A, it gathers speed and is moving fastest while passing through position A. We have learnt about two directions of movement, i.e., towards B or towards C. The term *velocity* is used to denote speed in a given direction. We can conventionally say that the velocity is negative when the movement is towards B and positive when it is towards C. When the displacement is maximum (B or C), the velocity is zero; when the displacement is zero (A), the velocity is maximum. Figure 27 shows the displacement and velocity curves of a pendulum.

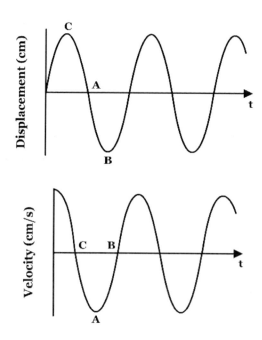

Figure 27. The displacement and velocity curves of pendulum bob.

In the above examples, a simple harmonic motion is referred as a cycle as repetitive movements are performed. However, simple harmonic motion is equivalent to circular motion which can be projected on a straight line. Figure 28 shows a circle whose center is the point O and the radius is of the length r. Imagine a point P moving round the circle at a perfectly uniform rate in an anticlockwise direction. It goes round and round the circle and because the speed is constant, the same time is required for each circle of

Bases of Speech and Language 65

movement. We shall start with position A on the horizontal axis of the circle. The point climbs up towards position marked C and then moves down to A'- B- and back to A. The distance that P has travelled at any given instant will depend on the angle travelled. A full circle is 360° and each quarter is 90°. So, when P reaches C the angle travelled is 90°, at A' it is 180°; at B it is 270°. Let us see how we can represent this angular motion. Assume that P has left A and reached P1 through an angle of 30^0. From this position drop a perpendicular line to the horizontal diameter of the circle the length of which is represented as p1 in Figure 28.

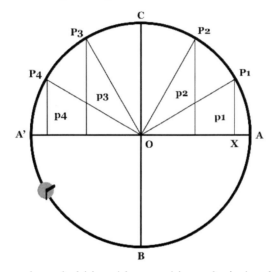

Source: http://www.pbs.org/opb/circus/classroom/circus-physics/pendulum-motion/.

Figure 28. Motion of point P on the circumference of a circle.

The distance from P to the center of the circle, O, is the radius r. The ratio p/r is the trigonometrical ratio called the sine of the angle at the center of the circle, i.e., in this example 30^0. Actually, you can take a ruler and measure the length of p1 and r. However; we can read the value of sine of 30^0 from mathematical tables which is equal to 0.5. If you go to P2 the angle is 60^0; again, drop a perpendicular line to the horizontal diameter of the circle the length of which is represented as P2 in Figure 28. Now sine of 60^0 is 0.87. When P reaches position C it has traversed 90^0 and sine 90^0 is equal to 1.0. The sine of the second quarter i.e., at P3 and P4 are equal to those for the first quarter; sine 120^0 = sine $60^{0;}$ sine 150^0 = sine 30^0 and so on. At position A' the perpendicular disappears or the value is zero and hence the sine is also equal to zero. For motion in the direction of B negative values are assigned. Based on the sine values we can plot a graph as shown in Figure 29.

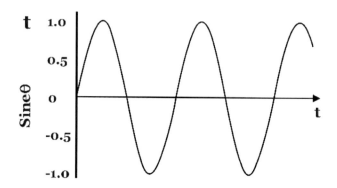

Figure 29. Graph of the sines of angles from 0^0 to 360^0.

We can now plot a graph showing the change in the sine of the angle traversed as time passes. For this, first of all we have to decide on the period for one cycle. Remember that equal angles are gone through in equal intervals of time. Let us take an example of period = 10 ms (F0 = 100 c. p. s.). Let us label the angle at any instance as θ. As said earlier we have to look up the sines in a table and assign to θ as many values as it is convenient to plot the graph. Remember to keep constant increments in the table. Let us take 10 steps from 0^0 to 90^0 and these will serve as the four quadrants of the circle. The sine θ would be as in Table 4.

Table 4. Sines of angles from 0^0 to 90^0

θ (Degrees)	0	9	18	27	36	45	54	63	72	81	90
Sine θ	0	0.16	0.31	0.45	0.59	0.71	0.81	0.89	0.95	0.99	1.00

X-axis on the graph would be time and Y-axis would be divisions between 0 and 1. The resulting graph would be the same as in Figure 29. By

Bases of Speech and Language 67

plotting the sines of angles from 0^0 to 360^0, you will arrive at the shape of a sine wave which is the same as the waveform of the vibration of a tuning fork or a pendulum. In this example we considered a frequency of 100 c.p.s. If we have 200 c.p.s., we would have a smaller circle as the radius would be small. However, the sines will remain unchanged.

Assume that you have two tuning forks; you have struck one and struck the second tuning fork after 2.5 ms. The prong of the second tuning fork will start moving from position A after 2.5 ms later than that of the first tuning fork. Also assume that the amplitude of vibrations of the two tuning forks is the same. When the first tuning fork has reached the position C on the circle, the second will be at position A (90^0 difference). This time difference measured in terms of angle separating two vibratory movements is termed *phase difference*. Figure 30 shows two sine waves with 90^0 difference of phase. When the time difference between two tuning fork vibrations is 5 ms, then it would be 180^0 out of phase. Figure 31 shows two sine waves with 180^0 difference of phase.

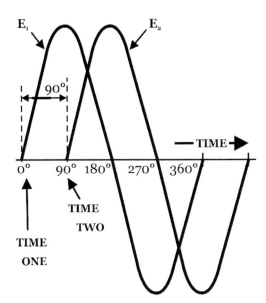

Source: https://www.physics.uoguelph.ca/tutorials/shm/phase0.html.

Figure 30. Two sine waves with 90^0 difference of phase.

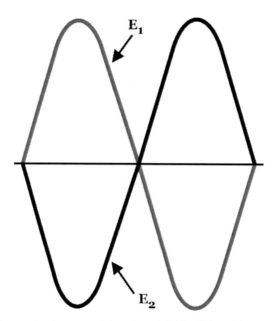

Source: https://www.physics.uoguelph.ca/tutorials/shm/phase0.html.

Figure 31. Two sine waves with 180^0 difference of phase.

Till now we learnt the simplest type of vibration represented as a sine wave. The resulting sound is called pure tone. Other examples of pure tones are whistle (sometimes) and may be low frequency notes. However, in nature sine waves are generated very rarely. Most of the sounds that we hear are *complex tones*. The wave of a complex tone is a complex wave. You have seen, in Figures 30 and 31, two vibrations with the same frequency but with a phase difference. If you listen to this sound carefully you will notice that it is louder than the single wave i.e., the amplitude is higher. However, we don't notice any pitch difference. This increase in amplitude is due to the fact that sine waves can be added together. Try plotting the waves on a graph with time on X-axis and displacement on Y-axis. You can literally add the displacement of two waveforms. Figure 32 shows the addition of two sine waves with 90^0 difference of phase. (See http://www.acs.psu.edu/drussell/demos/superposition/superposition.html for a demonstration).

Bases of Speech and Language 69

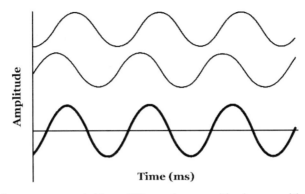

Source: http://www.acs.psu.edu/drussell/demos/superposition/superposition.html.

Figure 32. Addition of two sine waves with 90^0 difference of phase.

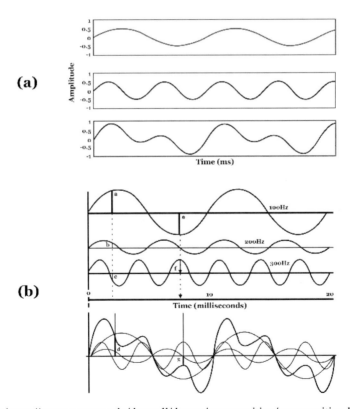

Source: https://www.acs.psu.edu/drussell/demos/superposition/superposition.html.

Figure 33. (a) Addition of two sine waves with different frequencies, (b) addition of waveforms with 3 different frequencies.

70   *S. R. Savithri*

You can do it yourself. Take a ruler and measure the values of displacement of two waveforms at each time instant. Algebraically add them and plot the waveform. This was an example of two sine waves with same frequency. Consider adding two sine waves with different frequencies. The waveform will be as in Figure 33.

2.5. Physical Properties of the Vibrating System – Elasticity, Inertia, Damping

Recall the movement of the tuning fork. When the fork was struck, the prong is pushed out of the resting position, to which it tries immediately to return. The vibration is resulting out of the property to return to its original / resting position. This tendency to resist being pushed out of shape and to return as rapidly as possible to the resting position is the result of *elasticity*. Materials vary widely in elasticity. For example, when a ball is dropped to the floor, it is momentarily pushed out of the shape; i.e., the part in contact with the floor is flattened and the elasticity of the ball makes it to retain its shape. The distortion of the material and the compression of the air inside the ball provide it with a restoring force which makes the ball bounce. You can do a very simple experiment with a rubber band. Pull the rubber band, leave it and observe the band returns to the resting position. (Watch http://agpa.uakron.edu/p16/video-ballbounce.php for a ball bouncing experiment).

Vibratory movements involve much more than elasticity. You have observed that the prong of the tuning fork overshoots the resting position (from B to C position via A position). This depends on the mass of the vibrating body. It is the mass that tends to resist movement when it is still and to continue movement once it is in motion. This is termed *inertia*. Vibratory movements are due to elasticity and inertia. Both these bring about repeated cycle of movements. The strength of the forces at work is determined by the distance from the rest position that is in this example the displacement of the prong. Newton's first Law of Motion states that "An object at rest stays at rest and an object in motion stays in motion with the

Bases of Speech and Language 71

same speed and in the same direction unless acted upon by an unbalanced force." Objects tend to "keep on doing what they're doing." It is the natural tendency of objects to resist changes in their state of motion, which is described as *inertia*.

No vibratory movement can continue indefinitely. Also, the amplitude of vibration should decrease as time goes on. The time taken for the cessation of vibration depends on the initial supply of energy. This energy is partly used in overcoming physical forces that oppose the movement (frictional force). For example, if you strike a tuning fork with a moderate blow it may continue to vibrate for about a minute. Assume you are giving a blow to wooden table with the same force; the vibration of the table dies down within a second. In the first instance you will hear a sound and in the second no sound is heard. The sound dies down very fast when you strike the table. The difference between these two is the difference in *damping*. The tuning fork has very little damping and the table has high damping. Damping refers to the property by which vibratory movements are reduced in amplitude / damped down. Figure 34 shows the displacement of a highly damped system.

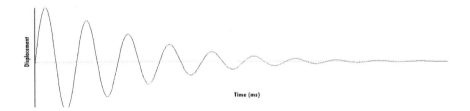

Figure 34. Displacement of a highly damped system.

Most of you will have attended a musical concert. Have you observed the tuning of background instruments before the singer starts the performance? When two tones are tuned to unison, it will present a peculiar effect. When these two tones are close in pitch, but not identical, the difference in frequency generates the beating. The volume varies like in a tremolo since the sounds alternately interfere constructively and destructively. As the two tones gradually approach unison, the beating slows down and becomes so slow that it is imperceptible. Therefore, a beat is interference between two sounds of slightly different frequencies and is perceived as periodic variations in volume. The rate of this variation is the difference between the two frequencies. (See http://en.wikipedia.org/wiki/Beat_(acoustics) for a demonstration). Figure 35 shows two waveforms with slightly different frequency and the beat produced by them.

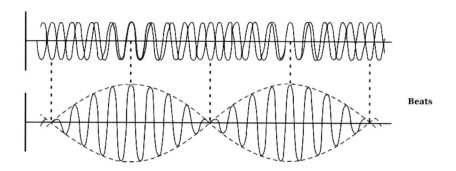

Figure 35. Two waveforms with slightly different frequency and the beat produced by them.

2.5.1. Propagation of Sound Waves – Transverse and Longitudinal Waves

We have already learnt about the tuning fork vibration and production of sound. If we are close to the tuning fork, we can hear the sound produced by the vibration of its prong. However, if we are far away, we can't hear it. Let us understand how the sound wave travels, prorogates and transmits. All of you will have seen the waves on water. If a stone is dropped in the water, you will see the ripples which are spreading from the center outwards in all directions as concentric circles. At the first instance we may think that the water particles have travelled from the center to the edge. But this may not be the case. Assume that a small cork or a piece of paper or a leaf, which is very light, was floating on the water before you dropped the stone in the water. You can observe that when the ripple reaches it, it moves rhythmically up, and down as successive waves pass through it. It does not move outward along with the ripples to outwards from the center. The particles of the water on the surface of the water move in exactly the same way as the cork; that is the individual water particle is moving up and down as in Figure 36.

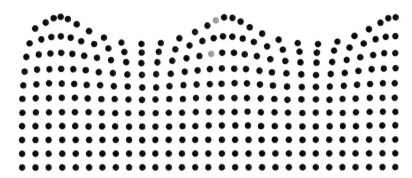

Source: https://www.acs.psu.edu/drussell/Demos/waves/wavemotion.html.

Figure 36. Individual water particles moving up and down.

Why are the water particles moving up and down? If so, how do we see the wave motion on the surface of the pond from the center outwards? We have already seen how the prongs of a tuning fork are moving when displaced from rest position, returning to the rest position etc. this property is shared by all kinds of particles we can think of whether it is metal or water (solid, liquid or gas). The water particles when displaced try to come back to the rest position. It has inertia, because of which the particles overshoot and go too far in the reverse direction. This sets up an oscillatory movement which is analogous to the tuning fork.

Assume that you have tied a rope to a post at one end and the other end is held in the hand, and you are doing a quick jerk upwards and downwards. This produces a wave motion in the rope which travels away towards the post. The particles are moving up and down; but as the particles are connected you see the movement as wave motion in the rope. Figure 37 shows the particle movement in a rope.

The particles of the rope in hand are forced into motion directly. Those at the successive points along the length of the rope are moving because they are connected with adjacent particles. They do so with a time lag which increases as you get further away from the hand. The movement of the particles of the rope is due to the inertia. The same principle is at work in the case of water particles also. It is now clear that no particle has moved towards the post where the rope is tried. The movement of the water particles from the center outwards is only because the water particles are connected together. The water particles are displaced at the point where the stone is dropped and it is transmitted from one particle to another, causing a vertical movement of the water particle and the wave motion in all directions outward.

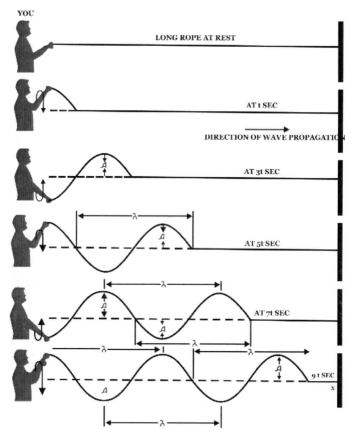

Source: http://physics.doane.edu/hpp/Resources/Fuller3/pdf/F3Chapter_16.pdf.

Figure 37. Propagation of a wave along a rope.

Observe the wave motion in Figures 36 and 37. The waves move from left to right horizontally, but the particles are moving up and down. The

Bases of Speech and Language

direction of particle movement is in right angle to the direction in which the wave is travelling. Such a motion is called a *transverse wave*. The movement of water particles as in Figure 36 almost resembles the sine wave, though not audible. Transverse waves can be set up on the surface of a liquid or in some solids as in the case of the rope. However, they can't be set up in gas and therefore the transmission of sound in air, which is the concern, will be different.

In the transverse wave the particle movement was in right angle to the direction in which the wave is travelling. As an alternative to this, there is another kind of movement. Imagine hitting a table on the side with a hammer as in Figure 38. The movement of the particles will be as in Figure 39.

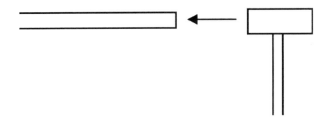

Figure 38. Illustration of a hammer hitting the table on the side.

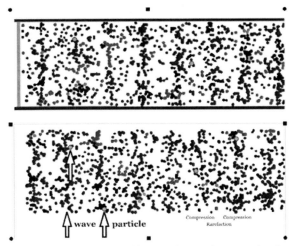

Source: https://www.acs.psu.edu/drussell/Demos/waves/wavemotion.html.

Figure 39. Particle movement when a hammer is hit on the side of a table.

In this case, the particle displacement is parallel to the direction of wave propagation. The particles do not move down the table with the wave; but simply oscillate back and forth about their individual equilibrium positions. Such a motion is termed as *longitudinal wave*. (Watch http://www.acs.psu.edu/drussell/demos/waves/wavemotion.html for a demonstration).

Figure 40. Illustration of transverse (table hit on the top by a hammer) and longitudinal (table hit on the side by a hammer) waves.

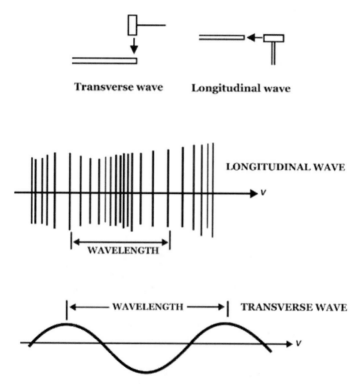

Source: http://physics.doane.edu/hpp/Resources/Fuller3/pdf/F3Chapter_16.pdf.

Figure 40. Longitudinal and transverse waves.

In a longitudinal wave consider particle number 1, which is next to the prong (row A in Figure 41). This is displaced to the right and left of the resting position as shown in row B in the Figure 41. Air particles affect each other when they move, just as the particles of water and rope did, but in a special way. When particle 1 moves to the right side it comes close to particle number 2 which is now forced to move up on particle number 3 which moves up on particle number 4 and so on as in row C. This crowding together of particle is termed compression and during this minute there is a rise in air pressure. With the passage of time a wave of compression travels to the right through successive particles. Meanwhile remember that there is a movement to the left side also. This creates more room to the right and creates a minute drop in air pressure so that particle 1 moves to the left. At this position the particles are spaced more widely than in the rest position which is termed rarefaction. A compression is succeeded by rarefaction (row D) which in turn travels to the right. The compressions and rarefactions are timed by the movement of the prong of the tuning fork and hence the frequency of the wave motion in the air is the same as that of the tuning fork. One move to the right and one to the left constitute a cycle of tuning fork motion. Hence one compression followed by one rarefaction will make up one cycle of the sound wave in the air. When the frequency of the tuning fork is 200 c.p.s., it will take 1000/200 ms i.e., 5 ms for the compression and rarefaction to pass through a given point in the air.

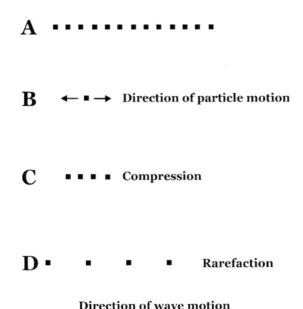

Figure 41. Particle motion in the path of a longitudinal wave.

Figure 42 demonstrates compression and rarefaction in a longitudinal wave. All sound waves reaching our ears arrive in the form of longitudinal waves.

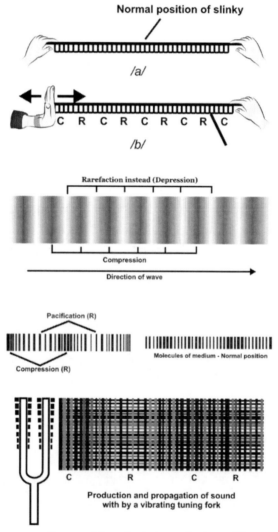

Source: http://www.excellup.com/classnine/sciencenine/soundCompressionRarefaction.aspx.

Figure 42. Compression and rarefaction in a longitudinal wave created by vibration of tuning fork.

Bases of Speech and Language 79

It was easy for you to visualize a transverse wave as a sine wave; but it is difficult to do so in a longitudinal wave. In a longitudinal wave, at a given point there will be a compression corresponding to the peak or crest of the sine wave. Sometime later, pressure at this point will have fallen to normal atmosphere pressure and will decrease further when a rarefaction is reaching, which is corresponding to the maximum negative value of the sine wave. Thus, a graph of the rise and fall of air pressure at a single point will yield a sine wave. Air pressure is represented on the Y-axis in arbitrary units, positive values indicating compression and negative values indicating rarefaction. Time is represented on X-axis.

Let us return back to the longitudinal waves. Assume you are sitting in a room and a tuning fork is struck by someone in the room. You hear the tuning fork sound because of displacement of air particles which is transmitted to the air particles next to your ear. It takes time for the air particle to travel. That is from the time the tuning fork is struck to the time you hear the sound. This can be very well understood by the example of lightening. You hear the sound of thunder after you see the lightening because sound travels slower than light. In other words, sound waves have some velocity. In air the velocity of sound is 340 m/s or 1240 km/h. Thus, a pistol fired 100 meters away from you would reach your ear by 0.29 s. The velocity of sound depends on the mass and spring. Velocity is high when the spring is stiff and vice-versa; velocity is low if the density (mass) is high. In air, though the mass is small, the springs are very slack and therefore the waves travel slowly. In contrary, in a steel bar, mass is high (dense material) and springs are stiff and hence the waves travel faster. If you are standing in a railway station you can hear the train approaching earlier via the metal rails than via air. The velocity of sound in steel is 5000 m/s, that is more than 14 times that in air.

We shall also look into the concept of wavelength. The wavelength of a sinusoidal wave is the distance between consecutive crests or troughs and designated by (λ). It is a measure of the distance between repetitions of a shape feature such as two alternate peaks, valleys, or zero-crossings as shown in Figure 43.

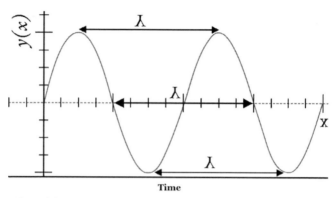

Source: http://en.wikipedia.org/wiki/Wavelength.

Figure 43. Wavelength represented by peak to peak or crest to crests or zero crossings.

The wavelength of a 100 c.p.s. tone will be 1000/100 = 10 ms. That of 200 c.p.s. will be 1000/200 = 5 ms and so on (1000 represents 1000 ms or 1 second).

2.5.2. Absorption, Reflection of Sound

We have already learnt that a wave propagating itself through a medium involves particle interaction; one particle applies a push or pull on its adjacent particle, which causes a displacement of that particle from the equilibrium or rest position. As one observes a wave traveling through a medium, a crest is seen moving along from one particle to another. This crest is followed by a trough that is in turn followed by the next crest. This sine wave that is seen traveling through a medium is sometimes referred to as a *traveling wave*. We also learnt about the frequency of the travelling wave. Now let us learn about another important property of the travelling wave, namely the amplitude. The amplitude depends upon several factors. First of all, it depends on the amount of energy available for conversion in to sound. For example, the amplitude of vibration of a tuning fork or a swing is largely dependent upon the strength of the blow with which it is struck. The tuning fork or the swing goes on vibrating/ moving till the energy supplied is used up and after the energy supplied is used up the body ceases to vibrate/ move.

We shall recall Figure 37 which depicted movement of a rope when tied to a pole at one end. In this example, the movement of the hand started a

Bases of Speech and Language 81

wave motion into the stretched rope which travelled towards the post to which it was tied. Here the total energy available will be dependent upon the force used and the distance through which the hand travelled. This energy will be used in moving the particles of the rope and will also determine the amplitude of the motion. If the rope is long and little force is applied, the wave motion will continue for only the first few meters of the rope and the amplitude will die down rapidly like the damped wave illustrated in Figure 34. On the contrary, if the rope is short and the force applied is more, the wave motion will continue throughout the rope to reach the post and the amplitude will be high. We already learnt that the first particle will push the second and so on when the wave motion starts. What will happen when the last particle of the rope tied to the pole is trying to push the next particle? There is no next particle of the rope and this last particle should push the post which is not possible. As a result, the wave will start travelling back along the rope or there will be *reflection* of the wave motion.

The reflected wave will travel as long as the original supplied energy is left to move the rope particles. This wave provides an example of visible reflection. In a similar way, when sound travels it encounters all kinds of obstacles and it is reflected from these obstacles. The echoes you hear from the hills or in a building are examples of reflection of sound. A sound will travel towards the hill and reflected which reaches our ear after some time. If there is more than one obstacle on the way of the sound wave, we may hear more than one echo at different times because these obstacles may be at different distances from the sound. In all cases the echo is weaker than the original sound. This means that the amplitude of the reflected wave is less than the original wave. This has to happen as the energy available is being used up as each particle pushes the adjacent. The term echo is generally used in instances where there is a time difference between the original and the reflected sound. The same phenomenon occurring in small rooms or concert halls is different in that there is an overlap of the outgoing and reflected sound as the distance the sound has to travel is not much. In this case the reflection of sound is referred to as *reverberation.* The amount of reverberation can be modified in various ways. The furniture, people, carpets etc. absorb sound energy.

The *absorption and reflection* of sound energy is influenced by the relation between the wavelength of a given sound and the size of the obstacle which it encounters. In general, a sound wave will be reflected if the obstacle it meets is larger than its wavelength and will be absorbed if it is smaller.

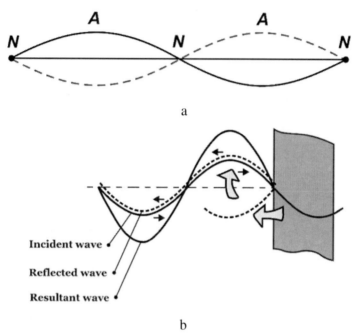

Source: http://hyperphysics.phy-astr.gsu.edu/hbase/Waves/standw.html.

Figure 44. Standing wave.

Now let us understand another case of sound reflection. Imagine an empty small room (4 m long) with very smooth and rigid walls. Set a tuning fork (515 c.p.s.) into vibration in the middle of the room. Sound waves travel out in all directions from the tuning fork, but for this purpose let us consider only one direction from the prong to the wall of the room. The frequency of vibration of tuning fork is 515 c.p.s. and hence the wavelength (λ = C/f, where C is the velocity of sound i.e.340 meters per second, and f is the frequency of the vibrating body) must be 34000/515 = 66 cm. Leave out some short distance in the middle of the room for the vibrating tuning fork. As the walls of the room are rigid the sound will be reflected, and the

Bases of Speech and Language

amplitude of the reflected sound is not very different from the original sound. Therefore, the wavelength of the reflected wave will also be 66 cm. There are two waves, one from the tuning fork and another from the wall in the opposite direction. The effect of these two-wave motion will be added together algebraically resulting in a wave shown as a continuous wave. Such waves are termed *standing waves*. Figure 44 illustrates a standing wave. Point A in the figure (a) refers to antinodes (maximum particle motion) and point N refers to nodes (no particle motion).

The distance between successive nodes and successive antinodes is half wavelength. In the room, there would be many frequencies whose half wavelength would fit an exact number of times into the distance between the source and the wall. The same thing holds for a stretched string. When a string is set to vibrate, many different standing waves occur in the course of vibration. Such standing waves fit exactly into the length of the string, that is each standing wave fit exactly into the length of the string; each must have nodes at the bridge (provided it is stopped by a finger) and at the nut (provided it is not stopped by a finger). The patterns of such standing waves that satisfy the requirement is shown in Figure 45. Here, the first wave involves the whole length of the string with a node at each end only (fundamental mode of vibration). The string length determines wave length of the sound. The second wave involves an additional node at the center of the string and hence it is vibrating in two halves. The string length determines 1/2 wave length of the sound. There are 4 nodes in the third wave and hence it is vibrating in 3 halves (1/3 wave length) and so on.

Each standing wave pattern is termed a mode of vibration. The string vibrates simultaneously in a number of different modes, that is, over its full length, in halves, in thirds etc. The frequencies thus produced will be multiples of the fundamental. For example, if the frequency is 100 cps in the first or the fundamental mode of vibration, then it is 200 cps in the second, 300 cps in the third and so on. These series of frequencies are known as *harmonic series*. The frequency at the fundamental mode of vibration is called the *fundamental frequency*, 100 cps in this example. The second harmonic is 200 cps, the third 300 cps and so on. This is a *complex sound* with the fundamental and its harmonics. Each mode of vibration is a sinusoidal and when combined they form a complex sound.

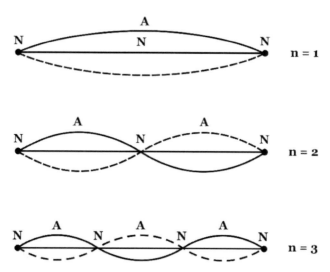

Source: https://hemantmore.org.in/science/physics/vibration-string/3151/.

Figure 45. Different modes of vibration in a string.

This example has a lot of bearing on speech sounds. Like the string instrument the vocal tract has a column of air and vibrating vocal folds. The relative amplitude of the fundamental and harmonics determines the sound quality. Two sounds may have the same frequency but may differ in quality because of the difference in the relative amplitude of the fundamental and harmonics.

2.5.3. Free and Forced Vibration

Till now we learnt about sounds that are produced by applying force to a vibrating body. As examples we have seen tuning fork, string etc. The force is applied only once, and such wave motions are the result of *free vibration*. A system which performs free vibrations will oscillate at its natural frequency or fundamental frequency. On the other hand, assume that you have struck a tuning fork and held it on a table top. The foot rises a little when the prongs are wide apart and descends when the prongs are close together. The foot of the tuning fork is pressed on to the table and is moving in time with the tuning fork; the table top also moves in time with the foot of the tuning fork. The tuning fork is now coupled to the table top. Now the top of the table starts vibrating and will continue vibrating till the force is supplied through the vibrating tuning fork. This is termed forced vibration. Figure 46 illustrates *forced vibration*.

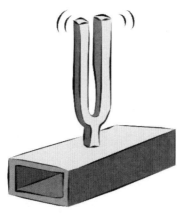

Source: http://www.physicsclassroom.com/class/sound/Lesson-4/Forced-Vibration.

Figure 46. Forced vibration of the table top in response to a tuning fork.

The amplitude of forced vibration will depend upon how tightly the two elements are coupled together. In speech, columns of air are forced to vibrate.

2.5.4. Resonance

Recall your 12th standard physics practical where in you held the vibrating tuning fork over the mouth of a jar with air column and poured water gently in to the jar. You reached a moment when the sound in the tuning fork rang loudly and clearly from the jar. This was because the air column in the jar was of the exact length to have a natural frequency which coincided with that of the tuning fork and thus has forced vibrations. In this example frequency of the tuning fork was fixed. The reverse may be done. Have a jar without water and find out the natural frequency of the air column by varying the frequency of the tuning fork. The natural frequency is that frequency when you hear the loudest sound. The amplitude decreases when the frequency of the tuning force is away from that of the natural frequency of the air column. The condition in which the frequency of the driving force is same as that of the natural frequency of the driven system is termed *resonance*. A curve relating the frequency of the driving force with the amplitude of the forced vibration is called resonance curve. Figure 47 illustrates resonance curves. It has two resonance curves; one which is highly damped and another lightly damped. Amplitude of the highly damped resonance curve is reduced compared to that of the lightly damped. High degree of damping means that there is relatively greater resistance for movement. An example of a highly damped system is table top or the nasal cavity. To summarize, greatest amplitude of forced vibrations will occur when resonance occurs or in other words when the frequency of the driving force coincides with the natural frequency of the driven system. A lightly damped system will have high amplitude and a narrow and sharp peak on the resonance curve. Because of this selectivity, such a system is said to be sharply tuned. On the other hand, the vibrations of a highly damped system die away rapidly, has relatively less amplitude and has a flat resonance curve.

Till now we learnt about the resonance of a single frequency as generated by a tuning fork. However, most of the sounds we hear are complex, in which case there are several frequencies. Therefore, the driving force contains several frequencies and its harmonics. What happens in this case? The principle of resonance remains unchanged. But, considering the earlier example of air column in a glass jar, and if the driving force includes the natural frequency of the air column, there will a peak output from the jar. It would appear as though the jar is selecting one frequency out of several frequencies. In fact, you can discover that the jar will also have other resonance frequencies. For example, if the natural frequency of the jar is 500 Hz, it will have resonance frequencies at 500 Hz, 1500 Hz, 2500 Hz etc. but, the amplitude of the forced vibration will decrease with increase in frequency. The principle of such multiple resonances in a column of air is the basis of speech. Figure 48 shows the multiple resonances of an air column in a jar.

Bases of Speech and Language 87

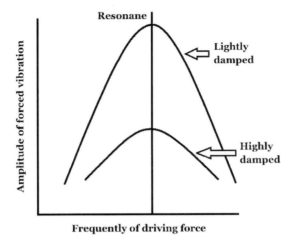

Figure 47. Resonance curves of two systems.

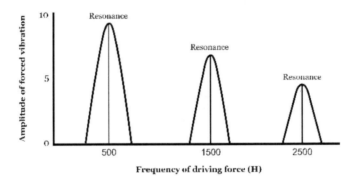

Figure 48. Multiple resonances of an air column in a jar.

2.6. Speech as an Acoustic Wave

The word resonance was used in several contexts and it is thought that it is good as it affords acoustic advantage. However, forced vibrations use up energy; a proportion of the driving force is spent in moving the resonating system and the remaining energy is the sound wave. Remember that you can't get more energy out of the whole energy that is put into it. Sounds can be amplified by electronic amplifiers in which we have additional energy of electrical power. Remember that resonators are not amplifiers and the energy they give out as sound waves is always less than the amount put into the system. We can reanalyze the illustration in Figure 48. We already leant that the driven system is responding with high amplitude of forced vibrations to driving forces at 500, 1500, and 2500 Hz. But, also remember that it is absorbing energy at other frequencies (for example, 501to1499, 1501 to 2499 etc.). When you consider resonators from this point of view you can call them *filters*. The acoustic filters reduce the amplitude of certain frequencies and allow energy at other frequencies to pass through with little reduction. The speech mechanism makes extensive use of this filtering function of resonators. Most speech sounds are complex tones and consist of a fundamental with all its harmonics. Therefore, description of speech sounds includes the frequencies that are found along with their amplitudes. This is referred to as a *spectrum* of the sound. The term spectrum is borrowed from optics which means consisting of various wavelengths of which light is composed of. A sound spectrum is analogous to this; but frequency is stated instead of wavelengths since sound travels through different media. To arrive at the frequencies and their amplitudes, one needs to break the complex signal in to its components. This process is called acoustic analysis. Figure 49 illustrates a sound spectrum.

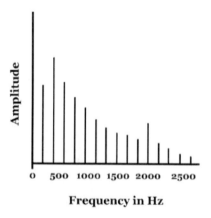

Figure 49. Illustration of a sound spectrum.

2.6.1. Speech Mechanism as Sound Generator

The sound waves of speech are the most complex to be found in nature. It has extreme changes very rapidly. Therefore, the speech mechanism must work in a very complicated way and in a variety of ways. Consider a stringed instrument like Veena or a Guitar. It has a vibrating source of sound which is coupled with a resonating system. Speech mechanism can be considered in the same way. The larynx and the vocal tract are analogous to the string and the resonating system. We have already learnt that the nervous system, the respiratory system, the laryngeal system and the resonatory system help in speech production.

3. ACOUSTIC THEORY OF SPEECH PRODUCTION

3.1. Acoustic Theory of Speech Production

According to the acoustic theory or the source-filter theory of speech production proposed by Fant (1960), speech is a product of source and filter or transfer function.

$$P = S * T,$$

where, P is the end product speech, S is the source and T is the transfer function of the vocal tract. Each of this is time and frequency dependent (Fant, 1960).

Figure 50 (a) shows the block diagram of source-filter theory. Vocal folds, the sound generator, are indicated as source. There are interconnected filter section each one representing a part of the vocal tract. Also, the coupling of the nasal cavity to the vocal tract is shown at the boundary of pharyngeal cavity and oral cavity. Figure 50 (b) is the quantitative treatment of speech production within a framework of electrical circuit theory. The cavities in front of the source are represented by four-terminal network. The output terminals are connected to the radiation impedance R. The network behind the source includes the source impedance and impedance of back cavities Z. the volume velocity through lips is represented by Is. Figure 51 shows the source and the filter in the vocal tract.

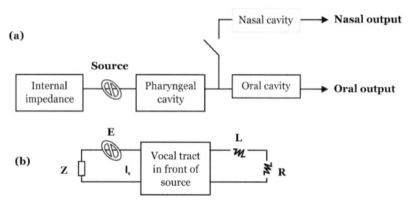

(a) Schematic representation of speech production with a glottal source
(b) Four-terminal network representation of non-nasal sound production irrespective of the sound location.
Source: Fant, 1960.

Figure 50. Speech production as a filtering process.

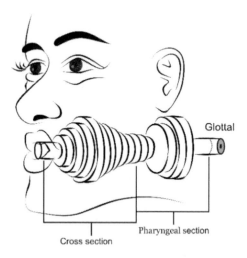

Source: https://www.google.com/search?q=source+and+the+filter+in+the+vocal+tract &tbm=isch&source=univ&sa=X&ved=2ahUKEwjPmLn1_NHiAhVBv48KHfZ5 ATkQsAR6BAgAEAE&biw=1440&bih=735#imgrc=IqdO0GqYMd82MM.

Figure 51. The source and the filter in the vocal tract.

One can think of source as equivalent to phonation and filter as equivalent to articulation. "In the above formula, S is an acoustic disturbance superimposed upon the flow of respiratory air and is caused by an object giving rise to friction or to a transient release or checking of the air stream and, in the case of voiced sounds, by a quasi-periodic modulation of the airflow due to the opening and closing movement of the vocal cords" (Fant, 1960). The basic property of the sound source is its periodicity expressed by the duration T0 or by the inverse of the F0 as shown below.

$$F0 = 1/T0, \qquad (1)$$

where, F0 is the fundamental frequency, and T0 is the time taken for one wave.

3.2. Source and Filter Characteristics

Voice source is characterized by its spectrum envelope S (f) which refers to all the frequencies and their amplitudes. All voiced sounds are quasi-periodic in nature. The various source possibilities according to Fant (1960) include

1) Voice source only
2) No source (Silence)
3) Noise source (one or several)
4) Mixed voice source and noise source

We shall learn about all types of sources. First of all, let us start with *voice source*. The respiratory muscles contract resulting in over pressure in lungs. The air from the lungs passes through the vocal folds as shown in Figure 52. The vocal folds open and close. Bernoulli's principle states that "for an inviscid flow of a nonconducting fluid, an increase in the speed of the fluid occurs simultaneously with a decrease in pressure or a decrease in the fluid's potential energy" (http://en. wikipedia.org/ wiki/ Bernoulli's_ principle). A bicycle commuter riding along experiences Bernoulli Effect. When a large truck passes the commuter, its speed creates an area of lower pressure and this draws in the surrounding air as it passes the cyclist. S/he feels as if s/he is being sucked toward the truck. In fact, s/he is! Another example can be found in the tap in a science lab. The flow is constricted in a very narrow nozzle. Above the nozzle is a small hole, which draws in air to create a vacuum in experiments. The vocal folds are also drawn in by the Bernoulli Effect. The intrinsic muscles of the larynx bring the vocal folds together, in the median position. The glottis is essentially closed off. Once they are closed, the air stream below the glottis creates a pressure against the closed vocal folds until they are blown apart. As the air rushes through the very narrow, constricted opening, it must accelerate to get through. This high-speed air, much like the truck in the example above, creates suction perpendicular to the direction of its flow and it draws the side of the opening in. Thus, the vocal folds perform closing and opening movements. In Figure 52, vocal tract is shown as a tube with one end open. One end of the tube is vocal folds and the other end is lips. Airflow from lungs is shown as stream; vocal folds are shown by vertical line. The opening and closing movement of vocal folds convert the stream of air in to puffs of air or in other words noise into voice which is shown as puffs in the oral tract.

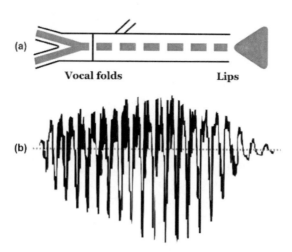

Figure 52. Schematic diagram of voice source (a) and waveform (b).

Bases of Speech and Language 93

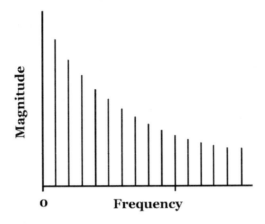

Figure 53. Illustration of source spectrum.

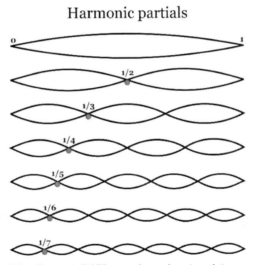

Source: https://en.wikipedia.org/wiki/Harmonic_series_(music).

Figure 54. Fundamental and harmonic partials of the voice source.

The vibration of the vocal folds generates a fundamental and harmonics which can be represented as source spectrum. Characteristics of the source spectrum are that the fundamental frequency has the maximum amplitude and the amplitude decreases as the frequency increases. The amplitude of the source spectrum decreases at a rate of -12 dB per Octave. Figure 53 shows a source spectrum.

The generation of harmonics is similar to that of a string explained earlier. F0 is generated at the fundamental mode of vibration. Harmonic partials are generated along with the fundamental as shown in Figure 54.

Let us assume that the F0 is 100 Hz. You can see the harmonics at 200 Hz, 300 Hz, 400 Hz, 500 Hz, 600 Hz, 700 Hz etc., which are multiples of the F0, in the spectrum. This is in the frequency domain. If we are visualizing the glottal waveform in the time domain, we can see a simple wave which is triangular in shape (Figure 55).

Glottal wave

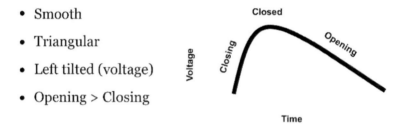

- Smooth
- Triangular
- Left tilted (voltage)
- Opening > Closing

Figure 55. A glottal waveform.

The glottis is represented by a high impedance termination of the vocal tract and therefore Fant (1960) defines the voice source by the pulsating airflow through the glottis. The waveform is saw-tooth shaped periodic time function as shown in Figure 56. Closing time is the duration for which the vocal folds are closing or coming to the mid line. Closed time is the duration for which the vocal folds stay in the mid line. Opening time is the duration for which the vocal folds are opening or moving towards the lateral side and open time is the duration for which the vocal folds are open or in the lateral side. Opening time is longer than the closing time in a glottal waveform. Figure 56 shows the opening and closing of the vocal folds.

Essentially the vocal fold is the first obstruction for the expiratory air, and it modifies the stream of air into puffs of air or voice.

Vocal fold vibration

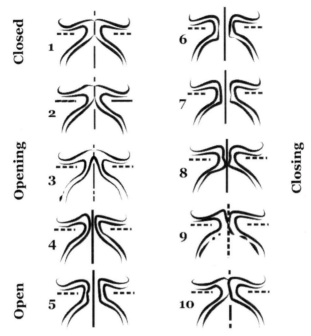

Source: https://voicefoundation.org/health-science/voice-disorders/anatomy-physiology-of-voice-production/understanding-voice-production/.

Figure 56. Opening and closing of the vocal folds.

No source or silence refers to a closed vocal tract or silence waveform as illustrated in Figure 57.

Silence

Figure 57. Silence waveform.

3.3. Noise Source

This refers to the primary acoustic disturbance within the vocal tract and is responsible for the generation of whispered sounds, aspirated sounds, frication, and plosives. In case of *whispered sounds*, the vocal folds do not vibrate and therefore the stream of air passes through the glottis unmodified. The modification, however, occurs at the glottis by the adduction of vocal folds which are adducted sufficiently to create audible turbulence or a hissing sound during exhalation. However, the articulation remains as in normal speech. Figure 58 shows the schematic diagram of a whispering sound.

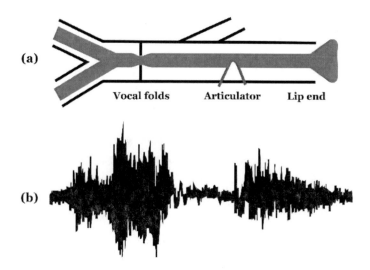

Figure 58. Schematic diagram of a whispering sound (a) and waveform (b).

Aspiration occurs when there is a larger opening of the glottis resulting in a strong burst of breath that accompanies the release of unvoiced plosives. Aspirated sounds or /h/ includes /kh/, /ch/, /t̯h/, /th/, and /ph/. *Frication* occurs when there is a relatively narrow constriction formed by the articulator in the oral cavity. The contraction of flow causes the air particles to accelerate which forms a jet of air at a high speed through the constriction. This is similar to water flowing through a hose pipe which is partially closed at the end of the water flow. This jet is associated with circulation effects

Bases of Speech and Language   97

and eddies, partially of a random nature. The place where these are created depends upon the flow and geometry including surface conditions. An obstacle hit by the jet of air will give rise to a turbulent source which is of greater intensity than a noise produced in a passage. An example of this can be the dental fricative where the upper incisors are the obstacle. The eddies around a free obstacle at low flow rates may give rise to a whistling noise of a quasi-periodic nature which is referred to as Aeolian tones or Schneidetone (Meyer-Eppler, 1953). "The tendency towards periodicity is likely to increase when the source is enclosed by a cavity resonator. At low flow rates the source will be influenced by one of the resonance frequencies of the cavity that determines the periodicity of the eddies. In such case, the impedance of the cavity system is low and resistive at a resonance frequency, and the flow has the effect of a negative resistance causing the system to oscillate. This is the case with either ordinary lip-whistling or whistling between the teeth. However, at increased rate of flow the periodicity can no longer be maintained, and the whistling changes into a random noise source. The source now rules the cavities" (Fant, 1960).

One of the important things to note in case of turbulence is the Reynold's number which is a dimensionless parameter proportional to particle velocity V cm/sec and to the effective width h cm of the passage. The constant $V = 0.15$ cm^2/sec is the kinematic coefficient of viscosity defined as the ratio of the viscosity coefficient to the density of gas. Reynold's number is expressed by the following formula:

$$Re = \frac{Vh}{V} \tag{2}$$

where, Re = Reynold's number, V = particle velocity, h = effective width of the passage, and V is a constant $= 0.15$ cm^2/sec.

In a relatively short constriction, the turbulent flow resistance is more influenced by the minimum area than by the length. Example of frication is fricatives. Figure 59 shows a schematic diagram of a fricative production.

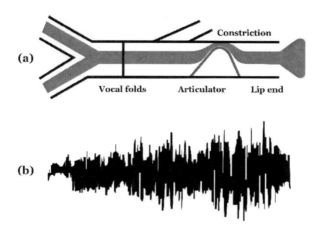

Figure 59. Schematic diagram of a frication (a) and waveform (b).

Another type of noise source is *transient* source. When the oral tract is completely closed by the articulator, the air is held behind; as the air pressure builds up behind the articulator, the articulator releases resulting in turbulent sound that are termed plosives. Owing to the finite opening time the step function is characterized by a spectrum envelope of - 6 dB/ octave. Plosives are produced in this manner. Figure 60 illustrates a schematic diagram of a plosive production.

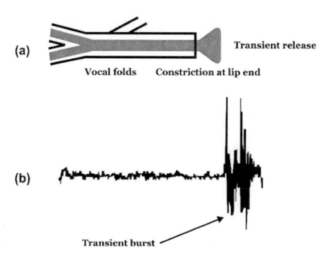

Figure 60. Illustration of a plosive production (a) and waveform (b).

Mixed source or Voice + Noise Source occurs when the vocal folds are vibrating but do not come to the mid position. This results in partial modification of air at the level of glottis; however, as the vocal folds are open to some extent the stream of air passes through it resulting in voice + noise source as in the production of /h/. Figure 61 illustrates the voice + noise source.

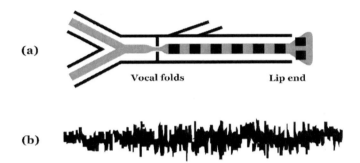

Figure 61. Illustration of voice + noise source (a) and waveform (b).

To summarize, we learnt about voice source, no source or silence, noise source, and voice + noise source. In case of voice source there exists a fundamental frequency with all its harmonics with a decrease of amplitude by -12 dB/octave. In case of noise source there is no fundamental frequency and the energy dips at a rate of - 6 dB/octave. Noise source can be aspiration, whispering, turbulence or transient. Usually voice source is used in the production of voiced speech sounds and noise source is used in the production of unvoiced speech sounds. Production of a speech sound may involve several noise sources; for example, transient and turbulence. We shall now move on to the filter or the transfer function of the vocal tract.

3.4. Filter Characteristics

Imagine pushing a swing. Each push should coincide with the motion of the swing or else you are likely to shorten its arc, or you may be knocked down to the ground. The frequency with which the swing completes a cycle during one second is the natural resonance frequency of the swing. This frequency is independent of amplitude. The natural resonance frequency of a swing would be higher when the rope of the swing is shorter. Everything that vibrates has a natural resonance frequency and the vibrating material has the maximum amplitude at its resonance frequency.

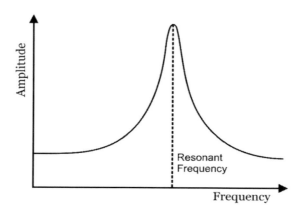

Figure 62. Illustration of resonance.

"Resonance is the tendency of a system to oscillate with greater amplitude at some frequencies than at others. Frequencies at which the response amplitude is a relative maximum are known as the system's resonant frequencies, or resonance frequencies. At these frequencies, even small periodic driving forces can produce large amplitude oscillations, because the system stores vibrational energy" (http://en.wikipedia.org/wiki/Resonance). "Resonance occurs when a system can store and transfer energy between two or more different storage modes (e.g., kinetic energy and potential energy in the case of a pendulum). However, there are some losses from cycle to cycle, which is termed damping. When damping is small, the resonance frequency is approximately equal to the natural frequency of the system, which is a frequency of unforced vibrations. Some systems have multiple, distinct, resonant frequencies" (http://en.wikipedia.org/wiki/Resonance). In simple words resonance occurs when the driving frequency of an oscillation matches the natural frequency, giving rise to large amplitudes. Figure 62 illustrates resonance.

Bases of Speech and Language 101

In a string fixed at both ends, the resonance frequencies are directly related to the mass, length, and tension of the string. The wavelength that will create the first resonance on the string is equal to twice the length of the string or in other words half wave is in the length of the string. Higher resonances correspond to wavelengths that are integer divisions of the fundamental wavelength. The resonance frequencies can be calculated by the following formula.

$$f = \frac{nv}{2L}$$

(3)

Where L is the length of the string, n = 1, 2, 3... (Harmonic in a closed end pipe), and v = velocity of sound in air.

Resonant frequencies depend on tension and length. It is increased with increase in tension and decrease in length. When the string is excited with an impulsive function (a finger pluck or a strike by a hammer), the string vibrates at all the frequencies that are present in the impulse. Those frequencies that are not one of the resonances are quickly filtered out—they are attenuated—and all that is left is the harmonic vibrations that we hear as a musical note.

A tube closed at one end is referred to as a closed tube. The tube has a fundamental frequency but can be magnified to produce other higher frequencies or notes. These frequencies can be tuned by using different degrees of conical taper. A closed tube resonates at the same fundamental frequency as an open tube twice its length or one fourth of the frequency wavelength. In a closed tube, a node, a point of no vibration, always appears at the closed end and if the tube is resonating, it will have an antinode, or point of greatest vibration at the Phi point (length X 0.618) near the open end.

By overblowing a cylindrical closed tube, a note can be obtained that is approximately a twelfth above the fundamental note of the tube. This is described as one-fifth above the octave of the fundamental note. For example, if the fundamental note of a closed tube is C1, then over blowing the pipe gives G2, which is one-twelfth above C1.

In other words, we can say that G2 is one-fifth above C2 — the octave above C1. Adjusting the taper of this cylinder for a decreasing cone can tune the second harmonic or overblown note close to the octave position or 8th. Opening a small "speaker hole" at the Phi point, or shared "wave/node" position will cancel the fundamental frequency and force the tube to resonate at a 12th above the fundamental. This technique is used in a Recorder by pinching open the dorsal thumb hole. Moving this small hole upwards, closer to the voicing will make it an "Echo Hole" (Dolmetsch Recorder Modification) that will give a precise half note above the fundamental when opened (http://en.wikipedia.org/wiki/Acoustic_resonance#cite_note-Jaap-5). The resonances of a closed tube can be calculated as follows:

$$f = \frac{nv}{4L} \qquad (4)$$

where "n" is an odd number (1, 3, 5...), L is the length of the tube and v is the velocity of sound in air (which is approximately 340 meters per second at 20°C and at sea level). Figure 63 depicts the first three resonances in a tube closed at one end.

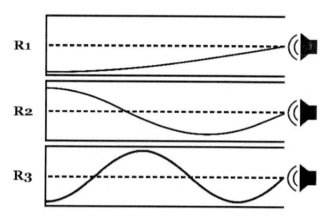

Source: https://en.wikipedia.org/wiki/Acoustic_resonance#cite_note-Jaap-5.

Figure 63. Illustration of the first three resonances in a tube closed at one end (R1 = First resonance, R2 = Second resonance, R3 = Third resonance).

In contrast, a tube in which both ends are open is referred to as an open tube. The tube resonates at many frequencies or notes. Its lowest resonance (called its fundamental frequency) occurs at the same frequency as a closed tube of half its length. An open tube will resonate if there is a displacement antinode at each open end. These displacement antinodes are places where there is a maximum movement of air in and out of the ends of the tube. Open cylindrical tubes resonate at the approximate frequencies:

$$f = \frac{nv}{2L} \qquad (5)$$

where n is a positive integer (1, 2, 3...) representing the resonance node, L is the length of the tube and v is the velocity of sound in air (which is approximately 340 meters per second at 20°C and at sea level). Figure 64 illustrates the first three resonances of the tube open at both ends.

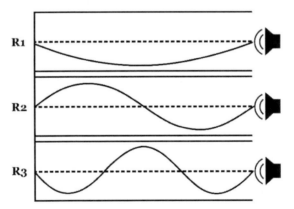

Source: https://en.wikipedia.org/wiki/Acoustic_resonance#cite_note-Jaap-5.

Figure 64. Illustration of the first three resonances in a tube open at one end (R1 = First resonance, R2 = Second resonance, R3 = Third resonance).

Now let us move to the production of speech. In case of speech production, especially vowel production, the vocal tract approximates a tube open at one end, which is at the lip end, and closed at the other, that is the vocal folds (during adduction). Vocal tract consists of the oral tract and the nasal tract. The length of the oral tract is about 17 cm and that of the nasal tract is about 12 cm. We have already learnt about the resonance frequency of such tubes open at one end. The frequency at which such a tube resonates will have a wavelength four times the length of the tube. Or, the first resonance frequency can be calculated by the formula $R1 = c/4L$, where, c = velocity of sound in air, and L is the length of the tube. Hence the first resonance frequency of the vocal tract would be 340 * 100/ 4 * 17 = 34000/ 68 = 500 Hz. Remember, the tube also resonates at odd multiples. Therefore, the second resonance frequency would be $R2 = 3c/4L$, that is 1500 Hz, and the third resonance frequency would be $R3 = 5c/4L$, that is 2500 Hz and so on. There are some differences between a rigid tube and the vocal tract. A tube is rigid, and the vocal tract is soft and has walls that can absorb energy. Also, unlike a tube, the vocal tract does not have uniform cross-sectional area. The cross-sectional area of the vocal tract changes from one location to another across the length which is illustrated in Figure 65. The vocal tract bends approximately at 90^0 at the junction of the oral cavity and the pharynx. None the less we shall consider the vocal tract as a tube.

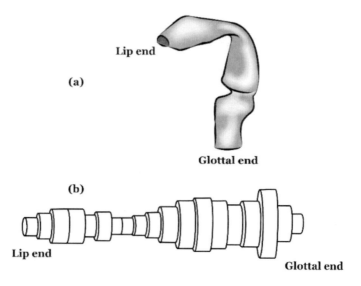

Source: Internet.

Figure 65. 3-D shape – MRI image (a) cylindrical sections (b) of vocal tract.

Vocal tract resonances are called formants, though there is some difference between the resonance and formant. The frequency of the first formant F1 is denoted by F_1, that of the second by F_2, the third by F_3 and so on. The vocal tract is considered as a filter (transfer function by Fant, 1960) which allows the resonance frequencies to pass through it and absorbs energy at other frequencies. If we consider it as a filter, it does exactly the work of a filter as illustrated in Figure 66. In this figure, 2 types of sieves are illustrated which filters unwanted particles.

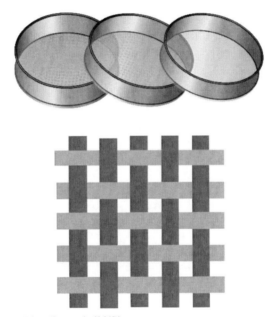

Source: https://en.wikipedia.org/wiki/Sieve.

Figure 66. Illustration of filter.

Now assume that the voiced source (fundamental and all its harmonics) are entering the vocal tract in which no articulation or constriction is made. Under this circumstance, as illustrated earlier, the resonance frequencies will be equal to those of a tube open at one end, lip end) and are 500 Hz, 1500 Hz, 2500 Hz etc. The energy at these frequencies are filtered or passed through the vocal tract and the energy at other frequencies is absorbed by the vocal tract. At the lip end, that is a product of source and filter, it will have peaks at 500 Hz, 1500 Hz, 2500 Hz etc. and dips at other frequencies. Let us represent the source, the filter and the product in frequency domain that is frequencies according to their intensities, which is termed a spectrum as illustrated in Figure 67.

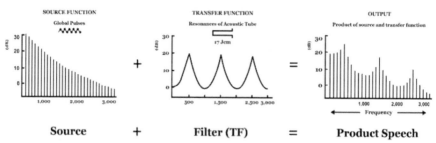

Source: https://www.google.com/search?q=Illustration+of+source,+transfer+function+(TF)+and+product+of+vocal+tract&tbm=isch&source=univ&sa=X&ved=2ahUKEwjtytD1xtbiAhVDOSsKHXBhAKEQsAR6BAgAEAE&biw=1440&bih=735#imgrc=ixMI2Ooa8sCaEM.

Figure 67. Illustration of source, transfer function (TF) and product.

Remember, these resonance frequencies are only for a vocal tract of length 17 cm. You know that the speaker can move his tongue, lips, and jaw creating various shapes of the vocal tracts. These shapes of the vocal tract bring in different shapes and volumes of the cavity which in turn change the resonance frequencies. So, you can consider the vocal tract as a variable resonator. The frequency selective transfer characteristics introduced by the process of multiplying the amplitude of each harmonic |S (f)| of the source spectrum by the value of the appropriate gain factor |T (f)| of the filter function at the frequency f:

$$|P (f)| = |S (f)| |T (f)| \tag{6}$$

To reiterate, vocal tract open at one end produces innumerable number of resonance frequencies such as 500 Hz, 1500 Hz, 2500 Hz etc. as illustrated in Figure 68. Also remember that the resonance frequency is inversely proportional to the volume of the cavity in that lower the volume higher the resonance frequency and the greater volume lower the resonance frequency. Therefore, smaller vocal tracts, as in children, will have higher resonance frequencies, and larger vocal tracts, as in adult males, will have lower resonance frequencies.

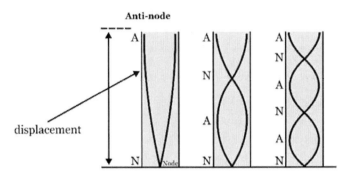

Source: https://www.google.com/search?q=Illustration+of+the+first+three+resonances+in+a+tube+open+at+one+end&tbm=isch&source=univ&sa=X&ved=2ahUKEwiNyPeGg9LiAhVFPo8KHeDDCiAQsAR6BAgAEAE&biw=1440&bih=735.

Figure 68. Illustration of resonances in the vocal tract (N = Node, A = antinode).

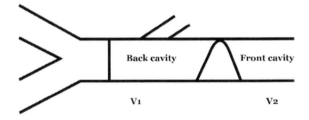

Figure 69. Illustration of vocal tract as back and front cavity.

These resonance frequencies occur when the vocal tract is at rest or without constriction. Now let us see what happens when a constriction is formed in the vocal tract. Assume that you are raising the tongue to produce vowel /a/. In such a condition a constriction is formed between the tongue and the palate and the tongue is approximately dividing the vocal tract into two cavities which can be called back cavity – behind the constriction – and front cavity – in front of the constriction as illustrated in Figure 69. The volume of the back cavity is represented as V1 and that of the front cavity is represented as V2 in Figure 69.

In such a condition, that is when there is a constriction in the oral tract, "frequency of the first formant is inversely proportional to the volume of the back cavity and the frequency of the second formant is inversely proportional to the volume of the front cavity, though erroneously" (Fant, 1960). The phrase *though erroneously* is used as the frequencies of the formants are influenced by several other factors like lip radiation, pharyngeal cavity, absorption by the walls of the vocal tract etc. In the production of vowel /a/, volume of the back cavity is low (small pharyngeal cavity) and that of front cavity is high (large oral cavity) resulting in formant frequencies at 700 Hz and 1200 Hz. Figure 70 illustrates the source, transfer function and product in the production of vowel /a/.

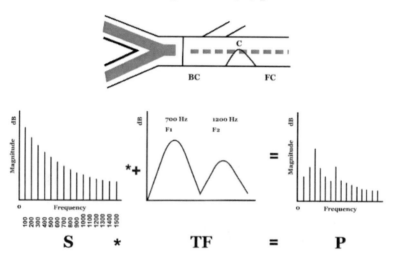

Figure 70. Illustration of source, transfer function and product in the production of vowel /a/.

In case of front high vowel /i/, as the constriction is around 4-6 cm back from lips' the volume of the back cavity is high (wide pharyngeal cavity) and that of front cavity is low (small oral cavity) resulting in formant frequencies at around 300 Hz and 2200 Hz. Figure 71 illustrates the vocal tract configuration, source, transfer function, and product in the production of vowel /i/.

Vocal tract configured for /I/ production

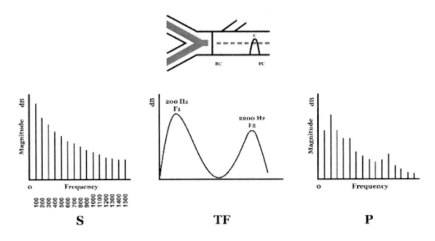

Figure 71. Illustration of vocal tract configuration, source, transfer function and product in the production of vowel /i/.

In the production of high, back rounded vowel /u/, the lip is rounded resulting in elongation of the vocal tract and thus lowering the formant frequencies. The raising of the tongue dorsum pulls the bulk of the tongue out of the pharyngeal cavity, enlarging and allowing it to resonate to the low frequency harmonics making the first formant. Also, the posterior constriction formed by the raised tongue dorsum and the protrusion of the lip lengthen the oral cavity and allows it to resonate to the relatively low frequency harmonics making the send formant. There are two constrictions formed in the production of vowel /u/; one at the back of the oral cavity and another at the lip end. For the purpose of a resonating tube, any constriction at the ends of the tube overrides the others and hence the primary constriction for the production of vowel /u/ can be considered to be at the lip end. Hence, the frequencies of the first two formants of /u/ occur at around 300 Hz and 900 Hz. Figure 72 illustrates the vocal tract configuration, source, transfer function, and product in the production of vowel /u/.

Vocal tract configured for /u/ production

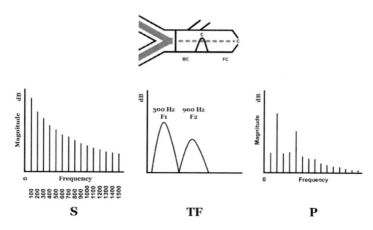

Figure 72. Illustration of vocal tract configuration, source, transfer function and product in the production of vowel /u/.

Figure 73 shows the articulatory positioning and area function for all three vowels and Figure 74 shows the formant frequencies arising out of the variable resonator – vocal tract – for three vowels.

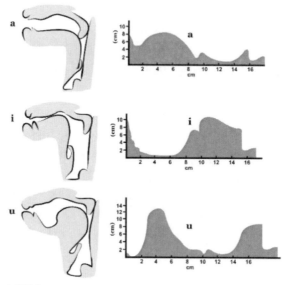

Source: Sreedevi, 2015.

Figure 73. Showing the articulatory positioning and area function for all three vowels.

Bases of Speech and Language 111

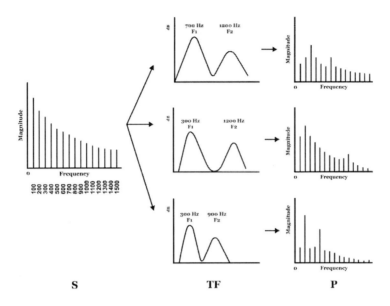

Figure 74. Showing the formant frequencies arising out of the variable resonator – vocal tract – for three vowels.

Thus, given the same source, the vocal tract, by changing its shape brings about a change in the resonance frequencies, which in turn determine the acoustic characteristics of speech sounds.

4. SOCIAL, NEUROLOGICAL, AND GENETIC BASES OF SPEECH AND LANGUAGE

4.1. Social Basis of Speech

An individual is integrated in to the society through communication and culture of a society is established and maintained through communication. As discussed, earlier speech and language are means of communication & speech is the best and universal mode of communication as hands and eyes are free during speaking. Speech is a medium of social control and emotions can be expressed through it. Through speech individuals are connected in a society. Speech may also isolate one group from another.

The belongingness to a group is strengthened through speech. For example, by saying "hello," "good morning" creates contact and relationship between people. In a public speaking the speaker has to bring forth the required response and behavior from the listener. The purpose of speech in a society is several. First of all, we speak so that the listener *understands* it. For example, a teacher in a class speaks or lectures for transfer of his knowledge to the students. That is his purpose of speaking is to make the students understand or add knowledge. Secondly, speech may also be used to *entertain or to divert*. Under such circumstance, the speaker is attempting to stimulate pleasant attitudes/emotions. He is not so much interested in imparting knowledge as in the case of a teacher above. The purpose of speech in this case is enjoyment, pleasure, amusement, relaxation or to remove negative thoughts of his listeners. Third, speech may be used to *influence belief*. For example, a leader may speak, and change believes of people. Fourth, speech may also be used to *influence action*. The action can be laughing, writing, voting or doing some other work like March past.

Group behavior is well known in social interactions and several types of groups like primary groups, play groups, work groups, family groups, what's App groups etc. Group refers to a number of persons who communicate with one another. Cooley describes a primary group as "those characterized by intimate face-to-face association and cooperation (Cooley, 1909). They are fundamental in forming the social nature and ideals of an individual. In a group the members meet, each member communicates with the other, and all members participate in the group. Communication and participation means speech at least in some groups." The effectiveness of speech is one of the problems of group dynamics as it is social interaction.

We have already learnt that speech is a means of social interaction. Once we know this, we also need to know the characteristics of good speech. First of all, speech should have a purpose and communicate the speaker's ideas to the listener. The voice quality should agreeable without breathiness, hoarseness, harshness, hypernasality, shrillness, muffling etc. Speech should be characterized by correct projection, articulation, fluency, prosody, appropriate selection of words and phrases.

Bases of Speech and Language

According to ancient Sanskrit literature *normal speech* was considered as one that which is sufficient, not redundant, not meaningless, not incoherent, not inconsistent, inoffensive, and with appropriate words. Good agreement between the speaker and the listener was also considered as an important aspect of normal speech, meaning that if speech is not understood by the listener it can't be considered as normal (Caraka Samhita). A *good speech* is that which has sense, is unequivocal, fair, pleonastic, soft, determinative, straightforward, agreeable, truthful, not harmful, refined, not too brief, not hard to understand, not unsystematic, not far-fetched, not redundant, not mistimed, and not devoid of an object (Mahabharata). In addition, if the words are adequate and not redundant it is said to be *excellent speech* (Nagarjuna in Upa:ya Kausalya Hr.daya). Clear speech was defined as that in which there is agreement between it on one hand and the speaker and the listener on the other hand. Speech, though clear to the speaker, if spoken without any regard to the listener, produces no impression (Mahabharata). It can be noted that the ancient Sanskrit scholars considered the speaker, the listener, the message and the situation and hence, the social basis.

4.2. Neurological Basis of Speech

4.2.1. The Neuron

The *neuron*, or nerve cell, consists of a cell body, dendrites, and an axon. Cell body is formed by a high concentration of potassium and low concentrations of sodium & chloride, compared to the fluids outside the cell body. The concentrations are reversed in the extracellular fluids, thus creating an electrical current for transmission of neural impulses. The **axon** carries neural impulses away from the cell body, and **Dendrites**, which are short projections, carry neural impulses to the cell body. The neuron can transmit neural impulses to other neurons, glands, and or muscles. Synapse refers to the juncture at which neural impulses are transmitted. Figure 75 shows a neuron.

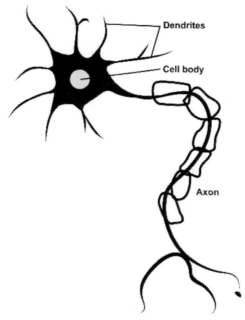

Source: from https://pixabay.com/en/axon-brain-cell-dendrites-nerve-1294021/.

Figure 75. A neuron with cell body, axon and dendrites.

Neuro chemical transmitters help in the transmission of neural impulses. Larger axons are insulated by Myelin, a fatty sheath, which increases the speed of neural transmission and reduces interference with the neural message. There may be about 100 billion neurons and 100 trillion synapses in the human nervous system.

As described in the previous paragraph, nerve impulses have a chemical component that underlies the electric potential of the cells. The charged particles or ions move through the cell membranes which results in action potentials. Nerve impulses activate the release of a neurotransmitter in a presynaptic neuron. This transmitter is the origin for the adjacent postsynaptic receptors to open an ion channel. When nerve cells conduct an impulse, positive and negative ions or membrane potential on each side of a cell membrane are unequal which is due to the unequal distribution of positively charged sodium and potassium ions and negative charged chloride ions and proteins across the membrane. The negative ions are highly concentrated inside the cell, and the positive ions are in higher concentration

Bases of Speech and Language — 115

outside the cell. Opposite ions attract, and identical ions repel. This forms an electrochemical gradient along the cell membrane, which is termed the cell's resting potential. The resting membrane potential is around –70 mV inside the cell membrane.

4.2.2. Nerve Excitation

The nerve cells are excited when there is a stimulus and forms a nerve impulse or action potential. The stimulus may be chemical or temperature change, electrical pulsing etc. As the negative ions are highly concentrated inside the cell, it is hyperpolarized, or it triggers a large spike. A change of at least 10 mV is required to trigger an action potential and depolarize a nerve cell. As the resting membrane potential is around –70 mV inside the cell membrane, a change which brings the cell interior from –70 to –60 mV is needed to trigger a nerve impulse or message.

4.2.3. Conduction of Nerve Impulse

Polarization is the basis of conduction of nerve impulses. Passive impulse conduction for a short distance takes place when sodium enters the cell membrane. By this, the interior of the axon becomes more positive than the adjacent area and the positively charged ions enter the cell membrane. In a similar way, polarization is the basis for exciting or inhibiting an impulse in the postsynaptic neuron. Excitatory postsynaptic potential is a lowered membrane potential in the postsynaptic neuron. This lowering of membrane potential creates a situation for a new impulse. The opposite happens in inhibitory postsynaptic potential.

4.2.4. Neurotransmitters

Neurotransmitters refer to chemical substances released at a synapse to transmit signals across neurons. They facilitate regulate brain mechanisms that control *cognition, language, speech, and hearing*, among other functions. The small-molecule transmitters include acetylcholine and the five monoamines derived from amino acids - dopamine, norepinephrine, serotonin, glutamate, and γ-aminobutyric acid (GABA). Large-molecule peptides produce longer-lasting effects. Largely neurotransmitters have

116   *S. R. Savithri*

more than one receptor type and may have different effects on different synapses. Because more than one neurotransmitter may be secreted by a single terminal bouton, it is not easy to identify a specific behavioral effect of a given neurotransmitter at all times.

4.2.5. Acetylcholine

Acetylcholine is the primary neurotransmitter of the peripheral nervous system (PNS) but is also important in the central nervous system (CNS). Actions of acetylcholine are slow and diffuse in the CNS, but succinct and clear cut in the PNS.

4.2.6. Monoamines

Dopaminergic projections are situated in the monostratal (midbrain and striatum) and mesocortical (midbrain to cortex) systems. Mesostriatal projections are dopaminergic cells from the substantia nigra to the putamen and caudate nucleus of the basal ganglia. Production and transmission of dopamine is reduced by the degeneration of the substantia nigra and is linked with Parkinson's disease.

Norepinephrine containing (noradrenergic) neurons is located in the pons and medulla, with most in the reticular formation. Noradrenergic neurons project to the thalamus, hypothalamus, limbic forebrain structures, and the cerebral cortex. Descending fibers project to other parts of the brainstem, cerebellar cortex, and spinal cord. Noradrenergic neurons are contemplated to be involved in generating paradoxical sleep and maintaining attention and vigilance.

Serotonin neurons are found at most levels of the brainstem, with terminals in the reticular formation, hypothalamus, thalamus, septum, hippocampus, olfactory tubercle, cerebral cortex, basal ganglia, and amygdala. It is concerned with overall level of arousal and slow-wave sleep. It also contributes to the descending pain control system. A feeling of well-being is associated with higher levels of this neurotransmitter and severe depression is thought to be connected with low serotonin.

GABA or γ-aminobutyric acid is the major neurotransmitter for the CNS and is the inhibitory neurotransmitter from the striatum to the Globus

Bases of Speech and Language 117

pallidus and substantia nigra, from the Globus pallidus and substantia nigra to the thalamus, and from the Purkinje cells to the deep cerebellar nuclei. Clinically, GABA is thought to be involved Huntington's disease.

4.2.7. The Human Nervous System

An overview of speech production already highlighted the human nervous system. It consists of the central, peripheral, and autonomic nervous systems. The CNS consists of the brain and spinal cord. The PNS consists of nerves, which are enclosed bundles of axons or long fibers. These nerves connect the CNS to parts of the body. There are two types of nerves, motor or efferent and sensory or afferent. Nerves that transmit signals from the brain to the other parts of the body are called motor nerves (for example movement of fingers) and the nerves that transmit information from the body to the CNS are called sensory nerves (for example sensation of pain). Spinal nerves serve both motor and sensory functions and are termed mixed nerves. The PNS has three separate subsystems, the somatic, autonomic, and enteric nervous systems. Somatic nerves are responsible for voluntary movement. The autonomic nervous system has sympathetic and parasympathetic nervous systems. We will review the areas of the human nervous system that are fundamental for speech and language.

4.2.8. The Brain

The brain consists of the cerebral hemispheres, the basal ganglia, the cerebellum, and the brainstem. The largest part of the brain is called the cerebrum. It is made up of the two cerebral hemispheres and the basal ganglia. The cerebral cortex covers the cerebrum and is composed of several important groves on its surface which are called sulci or fissures (grooves on the surface of the brain or spinal cord) and gyri (elevations or ridges on the surface of the cerebrum). Brodmann, a German neurologist, numbered 52 areas of the cerebral cortex, which remains as the universal standard till date and is referred to as Brodmann areas. Figure 76 shows Brodmann areas.

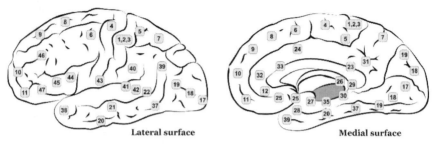

Source: https://en.wikipedia.org/wiki/Brodmann_area.

Figure 76. Brodmann areas.

4.2.9. Cerebral Hemispheres

The left and the right cerebral hemispheres are connected by corpus callosum which is a mass of white matter. The corpus callosum passes neuronal information from one hemisphere to the other. The left hemisphere has a different function than the right hemisphere. It is involved in language and analytical & logical aspects; whereas the right hemisphere is involved with perceptual, spatial, intuitive, and holistic aspects. For example, a lesion in a language area of the left hemisphere can result in aphasia, whereas a lesion in the right hemisphere can result in the patient's inability to draw information through inference which is arrived by a holistic and intuitive approach.

The longitudinal cerebral fissure, running from the front to the back of the brain, separates the two hemispheres. The cerebral cortex in each hemisphere is divided into frontal, parietal, temporal, and occipital lobes. The fifth lobe, the limbic, lies under the outer surface of the cerebral cortex. The *frontal lobe* is surrounded in the back side by the central sulcus and below by the lateral fissure. The central sulcus divides the brain into anterior and posterior regions. The precentral gyrus is within the frontal lobe and lies anterior to the central sulcus. It is also known as the *primary motor cortex*, and controls voluntary muscular movement on the opposite side of the body.

The neurons in the primary motor cortex are organized in a pattern of a person standing upside down. That is neurons responsible for motor movements in the face and neck area is closest to the lateral fissure, and neurons responsible for motor movements of the toes and leg are closest to

Bases of Speech and Language 119

the longitudinal cerebral fissure. The group of neurons responsible for the movement of the small muscles of the larynx, palate, tongue, jaw, and face are greater than to the arm or leg. Hence the number of neurons assigned for voluntary movement of a body part is not proportionate to its size. A lesion in the primary motor cortex within areas involving movements of the lips, tongue, or larynx can result in certain types of dysarthria. The premotor and supplementary motor areas are located in front of the precentral gyrus. These areas receive information from other regions of the brain, integrate, refine, and plan or program motor speech output. Broca's area is in the third frontal gyrus of the dominant hemisphere. Broca's area plays a major role in motor speech programming. It connects to other parts of the brain involved with speech and language. A lesion in Broca's area may result in apraxia of speech in addition to nonfluent aphasia.

The *parietal lobe* is bounded below by the back end of the lateral fissure and in the front by the central sulcus. The postcentral gyrus located in back of the central sulcus lies within the parietal lobe. The postcentral gyrus is a mirror image to the "motor strip" area of the frontal lobe and is the primary sensory cortical area ("sensory strip"). It has to do with the sense of temperature, pain, touch, and proprioception. Proprioception facilitates one to realize exactly where the individual parts of the body are in space, and the relationship of one body part to another. For example, the position of the tongue in relation to the other parts of the oral tract in the production of speech sounds can be sensed. The somatosensory cortex in the dominant hemisphere plays a role in speech motor programming, especially in the integration of sensory information in preparation for motor activity. Also, the somatosensory cortex in the right hemisphere helps maintain reasoning and decision making, emotion, and feelings, with a special emphasis in the social and personal domain (Damasio, 1994). The supramarginal gyrus and the angular gyrus are located in the parietal lobe of the dominant hemisphere. The supramarginal gyrus is responsible for the formulation of written language and probably for phonological storage. A lesion in this area can result in aphasia. The angular gyrus plays a major role in reading comprehension and a lesion in this area can result in aphasia with deep dyslexia.

120 *S. R. Savithri*

The *temporal lobe* is surrounded in the back by the front border of the occipital lobe and on top by the lateral fissure. There are three important areas in the temporal lobe of the dominant hemisphere - Heschl's gyrus, Wernicke's area, and the insula (or the Island of Reil) -. Heschl's gyrus or primary auditory cortex is the cortical center for hearing. It is responsible for appreciating the meaning of sound. A lesion in this area may result in auditory processing problems, resulting in auditory comprehension deficits. Wernicke's area or auditory association area is responsible for auditory comprehension and other language abilities. A lesion in this area can result in aphasia. The insula is visible when the two borders of the lateral fissure are pulled apart. The function of the insula is not clearly understood. However, a lesion of Insula may result in aphasia or apraxia of speech.

The *occipital lobe* is situated at the back of the cerebral hemisphere. It is bounded in the back by the longitudinal fissure and in the front by the parietal and temporal lobes. The primary visual cortex and visual association areas are situated in the occipital lobe. The primary visual cortex is responsible for basic vision and a lesion in this area can result in blindness. The visual association area is responsible for integrating and organizing incoming visual stimuli. A lesion of this area may result in visual perception problems, which in turn can influence reading comprehension.

The *limbic lobe* is on the medial surface of the cortex and contains the orbital frontal region, the cingulate gyrus, and the medial portions of the temporal lobe. It regulates emotions and behavior and a lesion in this system can affect prosody or suprasegmental or may be pragmatic abilities. Figure 77 shows the lateral surface of cerebrum and Figure 78 shows the superior view of the cerebral hemisphere.

The *association areas* connect the primary centers for motor, sensory, hearing, and visual functioning to other parts of the brain. They are responsible for higher mental functioning, including language, and are located in the lobes of each hemisphere. The *frontal association area* initiates and integrates purposeful behavior, planning and carry out sequences of volitional movement. The *parietal association area*, or somesthetic area, is responsible for the discrimination and integration of tactile information. The *temporal or auditory association area* is responsible

Bases of Speech and Language 121

for the discrimination and integration of auditory information. The *visual association area* discriminates and integrates visual information. A lesion in an association area of the dominant hemisphere can also lead to aphasia, as the connection between association areas is broken down.

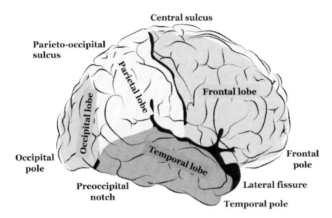

Lateral surface of cerebrum 4 lobes are shown
Source: https://en.wikipedia.org/wiki/Lobes_of_the_brain.

Figure 77. Lateral surface of cerebrum.

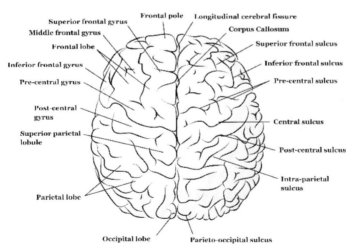

Source: https://www.slideshare.net/jeffarian/general-appearance-of-the-cerebral-hemispheres.

Figure 78. Superior view of the cerebral hemisphere.

The subcortical structures are called the *basal ganglia or basal nucleus which is* a mass of grey matter and lies deep within the cerebrum and below the cerebral cortex. It consists of the caudate nucleus, the Globus pallidus, and the putamen. Together these are called the *corpus striatum*. The basal ganglia controls and stabilizes motor functions, interprets sensory information which guides and controls motor behavior. Hence, a lesion in the basal ganglia can result in dysarthria.

4.2.10. The Cerebellum

The cerebellum is a tightly folded layer of cortex, with white matter underneath and is located at the base of the occipital lobe just behind the pons and the medulla. It has two hemispheres - right and left - which are connected by the vermis. These are most involved in speech control and helps in coordinating the skilled, voluntary muscle activity produced elsewhere by the connections to the spinal cord, cerebrum, pons, and medulla. A lesion in the cerebellum can result in dysarthria. Figure 79 shows a drawing of cerebellum.

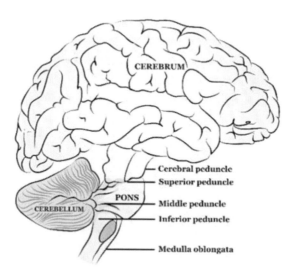

Source: https://en.wikipedia.org/wiki/Anatomy_of_the_cerebellum.

Figure 79. Drawing of cerebellum.

4.2.11. The Brainstem

The brainstem emerges as an upward extension of the spinal cord and pushes upward into the brain between the cerebral hemispheres. It consists of *the medulla oblongata, the pons, the midbrain* (mesencephalon), and two structures (diencephalon) called the *thalamus and hypothalamus*. The *medulla* consists of the nuclei for several of the cranial nerves and ascending and descending tracts to and from the cortex that are important for the control of speech production. The *pons* also has nuclei for several of the cranial nerves, major connections to the cerebellum, and other connections to the cortex which are important for speech production. A lesion in a cranial nerve important for speech can result in dysarthria. The *midbrain, thalamus, and hypothalamus* are a way station in the auditory and visual nervous systems and contain the synapses for vision and hearing. The *midbrain* also contains the substantia nigra, which is responsible for the production of the chemical neurotransmitter dopamine that helps in motor control and muscle tone. Thus, a lesion in the substantia nigra may cause dysarthria. The *thalamus* station for sensory information going to and from the sensory areas of the cortex. It has direct relationship with cortical language and motor speech systems. A lesion in the thalamus can result in aphasia. The *hypothalamus* controls some emotional behavior and helps in the regulation of body temperature, food and water intake, and sexual and sleep behavior.

4.2.12. The Spinal Cord

The spinal cord extends from the skull through foramen magnum, a large opening, down to the lower back. It is enclosed in the vertebral column with an H-shaped area of grey matter in the core of the spinal segment in a cross section. The grey matter has motor and sensory neurons. The ventral or anterior portion of the cord conducts motor neurons, and the dorsal or posterior portion of the cord conducts sensory neurons. There are 31 pairs of Spinal Nerves that are connected to the spinal cord. The spinal cord, through these nerves, sends sensory information (pain, temperature, touch, and vibration) from the receptor to the cortex for appraisal of the sensations. The spinal nerves send motor information from the CNS to the effectors. The spinal cord contains grey and white matter. The grey matter contains the nerve cell bodies, and the white matter contains the ascending and descending nerve axon fibers. Ascending tracts carry sensory or afferent information, and descending tracts carry motor or efferent information. Figure 80 shows a cross section of spinal cord.

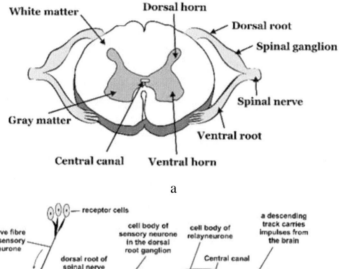

a

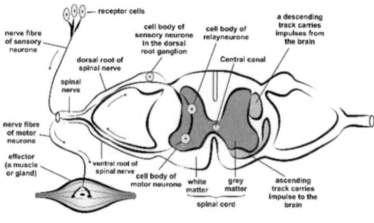

b

Source: https://www.google.co.in/search?q=Cross+section+of+the+spinal+cord&client=firefox-b-ab&dcr=0&tbm=isch&tbo=u&source=univ&sa=X&ved=0ahUKEwiiva2XstvWAhULN48KHZyJAT4QsAQIIJg.

Figure 80. Cross section of spinal cord.

Sometimes, a motor response can avoid going through the higher centers of the cortex for interpretation and use a shortcut known as the *reflex arc*. A receptor can respond to pain or temperature and send this information through a sensory neuron, which further sends it to the dorsal horn in the spinal cord. At this point, instead of going to higher centers of the cortex, the impulse can travel through an interneuron in the spinal cord to the ventral (or anterior) horn. From there, the impulse descends through the motor neuron and into the effector (e.g., muscles), the action of which will cause an instant action such as instant removal of hand from hot water or an electric shock. Different types of reflexes exist at different levels within the nervous system.

4.2.13. The Meninges

The brain and the spinal cord are protected and nourished by a system engaging the meninges, ventricles, and blood supply. Further, the hard bone of the cranium and the bony vertebral column protect the brain and spinal cord. Meninges are three membranes below the bone. The meninges has the *dura mater*, which is tough, the *arachnoid mater*, and the *piamater*, both of which are delicate. Space between meninges separates it and provides a cushioning effect. The space between the outer bone and the dura mater is termed extradural space. Below the dura mater is the subdural space. The subarachnoid space is located between the arachnoid mater and the pia mater and contains cerebrospinal fluid. Figure 81 shows the meninges.

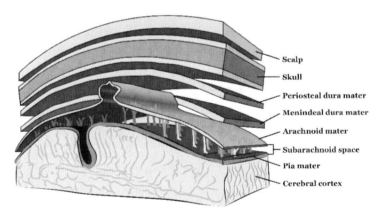

Source: https://www.thoughtco.com/brain-anatomy-meninges-4018883.

Figure 81. Meninges.

4.2.14. The Ventricles

Ventricles, four in number, are the network of cavities within the brain. There are two lateral ventricles, the third ventricle, and the fourth ventricle. They are interconnected by small canals and ducts. The choroid plexus within each ventricle produces cerebrospinal fluid which fills all the ventricles. The cerebrospinal fluid, through small openings in some ventricles, fills the subarachnoid space of the meninges. This fluid helps in the nourishment of nerve tissues, regulates intracranial pressure, removes waste products, and along with the meninges, cushions and protects the brain & spinal cord from physical trauma. The paired lateral ventricle is connected to the third ventricle through the intraventricular foramen or the foramen of Monro. The third ventricle is connected to the fourth ventricle through the cerebral aqueduct or the aqueduct of Sylvius. Congenital blockage of the cerebral aqueduct is associated with *hydrocephalus*. The fourth ventricle goes into the subarachnoid space via the foramen of Luschka and the foramen of Magendi. The cerebrospinal fluid flows into the brain and the spinal cord, and finally drains into the venous system for excretion through this ventricular route.

4.2.15. The Blood Supply

Blood is made of a liquid component the plasma, and solid components made up of red corpuscles, white corpuscles, and platelets. Red corpuscles are cells produced in the bone marrow and carry oxygen from the lungs to other parts of the body. For proper nutrition and functioning the brain requires oxygen and other elements carried by the blood. Cell death can occur, when the blood supply to the brain is stopped for five minutes or longer. Arteries carry blood away from the heart, and veins carry blood toward the heart. Capillaries connect the arteries to the veins. The heart pumps blood into the aorta, a major artery. Aorta branches off into four main arteries - two common carotid arteries one for each side, and the two common subclavian arteries one for each side. The two common carotid arteries ascend into the brain and divide into an internal carotid artery and an external carotid artery. The external carotid branch supplies the face area. The internal carotid branch further branches into the anterior and middle

Bases of Speech and Language 127

cerebral arteries. The *anterior cerebral artery* supplies the anterior and superior frontal lobes, corpus callosum, the medial surfaces of the hemispheres, and parts of the subcortical areas. The *middle cerebral artery* supplies most of the lateral surfaces of the hemispheres and parts of the subcortical areas. The two *common subclavian arteries* branches into *vertebral arteries* and ascend into the brain. The branches (one from each side) of the vertebral artery join together to form the *basilar artery*. The basilar artery ascends and branches into two *posterior cerebral arteries* which supply the inferior lateral surface of the temporal lobe, and the lateral & medial surfaces of the occipital lobe, parts of the spinal cord, medulla, pons, midbrain, and cerebellum. The union of the two internal carotid arteries and the two vertebral arteries in the brainstem forms the *circle of Willis*. A stoppage of the blood supply above the circle of Willis may cause brain damage than below the circle of Willis. When a stoppage occurs above the circle, alternative blood channels are not readily available, and this can lead to a cerebrovascular accident resulting in *aphasia*.

4.2.16. The Motor System for Speech

The neural motor pathways for speech control exist at all levels of the nervous system. It consists of the *pyramidal system and the extrapyramidal system*. The pyramidal system has the corticospinal tract and the corticobulbar tract that are responsible for skilled voluntary motor movement. The role of the pyramidal system is mainly facilitative.

The *corticospinal tract*, originating from the motor cortex or in the premotor cortex, controls skilled voluntary movements of the limbs and trunk. The precentral gyrus (motor strip area) of the frontal lobe, and to some extent, the premotor area of the frontal lobe and the postcentral gyrus (sensory strip area) of the parietal lobe are involved. The corticospinal tracts descend from the cortex to the internal capsule, a subcortical structure and converge. From there, the tracts further descend through the midbrain, the pons, and the medulla, and then to various levels of the spinal cord. Here they synapse with the spinal nerves of the peripheral nervous system. About 85–90% of the corticospinal tracts cross over to the other side of the body in to the upper medullary pyramids before reaching the spinal nerves. Hence it is named pyramidal system. A lesion above the crossover decussation point of the medullary pyramids may result in paralysis of the contralateral limb and a lesion below the crossover point may result in paralysis of the ipsilateral limb. The corticospinal tracts that cross over are called the lateral corticospinal tracts (85–90%), and those that do not cross over are called the anterior corticospinal tracts (10–15%). Figure 82 shows a schematic diagram of the pyramidal system in speech production, and the cranial nerves responsible for the innervation of the muscles used in phonation, resonance, and articulation.

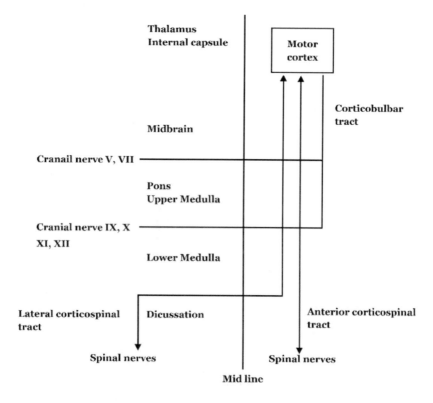

Figure 82. Schematic diagram of the pyramidal system in speech production, and the cranial nerves responsible for the innervations of the muscles used in phonation, resonance, and articulation.

The *corticobulbar tract* or *medulla* controls the skilled voluntary movements of the speech muscles, except those of respiration. The

Bases of Speech and Language   129

corticobulbar tract descends to the motor nuclei of the cranial nerves located in the pons and the medulla. It has several ipsilateral and contralateral fibers, and the crossover takes place at several levels of the brainstem. The corticobulbar tract produces bilateral innervation and therefore the majority of the midline structures work in bilateral symmetry. A unilateral lesion to the corticobulbar tract may result in a mild dysarthria due to assistance from the intact muscles of the other side.

The *extrapyramidal system* includes the indirect activation pathway and the control circuit areas. The *indirect activation pathway* has numerous short pathways originating from the cerebral cortex and ending in the spinal cord and in the cranial nerves. This pathway is influenced by the basal ganglia and cerebellar control circuits. It interacts with the corticospinal and corticobulbar tracts of the pyramidal system. The activation pathway (Duffy, 2005) helps regulate reflexes and maintain tone, posture, and other associated activities. It also helps the direct motor system in achieving the proper speed, range, and direction of specific muscular movements. A unilateral lesion in the indirect activation pathway can result in a unilateral upper motor neuron dysarthria; bilateral lesions can result in a *spastic dysarthria*. The indirect activation pathway also contains several tracts which are inhibitive in function. The *control circuits* consist of the *basal ganglia control circuit* and the *cerebellar control circuit*. These control circuits have direct contact with the cortex, with parts of the pyramidal system and indirect activation pathways, and with themselves. They give information and sensory feedback to the pyramidal system and indirect activation pathways regarding the posture, orientation in space, tone, and physical environment in which timed and coordinated muscular movement will take place. Motor disturbances related to the basal ganglia control circuit are called dyskinesias or involuntary movement disorders. The symptoms shown in hypokinetic dysarthria, associated with Parkinson disease, is a dyskinesias and symptoms shown in hyperkinetic dysarthria, associated with Huntington disease is a hyperkinesia, or too much movement. Incoordination and hypotonia are motor disturbances of the cerebellar control circuit. A lesion in the cerebellar control circuit may result in *ataxic dysarthria*.

130   S. R. Savithri

4.2.17. The Upper and Lower Motor Neurons

The *upper motor neuron* (UMN) pathways are the pyramidal system or direct motor system, and a part of the extrapyramidal system (or indirect motor system). The pyramidal system consists of the corticospinal tracts. These tracts send motor impulses from the cortex to the spinal cord, and the corticobulbar tracts, which further send motor impulses from the cortex to the cranial nerves located in the pons and the medulla. The indirect activation pathway, which is a part of the extrapyramidal system, sends motor impulses from the cortex to the spinal cord, the cranial nerves, and the corticospinal and corticobulbar tracts.

The role of indirect activation pathway to the cranial nerves involved in speech production is not very well understood. The UMN pathways activate the lower motor neuron (LMN). Damage to the UMN can result in a spastic paralysis, characterized by hypertonia (extreme tension of the muscles), hyperreflexia (an exaggeration of deep tendon reflexes), little or no atrophy (loss of bulk) of the musculature, and no fasciculations (fine muscle twitches). This may lead to decreased skilled movements, weakness, slowness, and reduced range of movement of the speech musculature. A bilateral UMN damage results in *spastic dysarthria*.

The lower motor neuron (LMN) or *final common pathway* (FCP) consists of the 31 pairs of spinal nerves and 12 pairs of cranial nerves. The LMN pathways are activated by the UMN pathways and they in turn send motor impulses to the muscles for movement. The spinal nerves transmit motor impulses to the limbs, trunk, and the muscles used for respiration. The cranial nerves send motor impulses to the muscles of the speech mechanism. A damage to the LMN may result in flaccid paralysis and is characterized by hypotonia, hyporeflexia, atrophy of the musculature, and fasciculations. This in turn results in weakness of the speech musculature. Lesions to the motor unit of the LMN can occur anywhere - in the cell body, in the axon leading to the muscle, at the neuromuscular junction, or in the muscle itself -. Bilateral damage to any portion of the motor unit results in a *flaccid dysarthria*.

4.2.18. The Peripheral Nervous System

The peripheral nervous system (PNS) consists of 31 pairs of spinal nerves and 12 pairs of cranial nerves. The spinal Nerves leave from the spinal cord and conduct sensory and motor impulses to and from other parts of the body. Each pair of spinal nerve has a dorsal (posterior) root that carries sensory messages through afferent fibers to the CNS, and a ventral (anterior) root which carries motor messages through efferent fibers from the CNS. The sensory messages (e.g., pain, touch, temperature) pass through the thalamus, and the thalamus transmits the messages to the sensory cortex (postcentral gyrus) for evaluation. The motor messages are sent from the CNS (corticospinal tracts) to the spinal nerves of the PNS, and they in turn send the message to the muscles of the limbs and the trunk. The 31 pairs of spinal nerves include 8 pairs of cervical nerves, 12 pairs of thoracic nerves, 5 pairs of lumbar nerves, 5 pairs of sacral nerves, and 1 pair of coccygeal nerves. Parts of the thoracic division are responsible for the abdominal and intercostal muscles, and parts of the cervical division form the phrenic nerves are responsible for the movement of the diaphragm muscle. All these muscles are involved in the respiration which is very important in speech production as air is the source of speech. Bilateral lesions result in weakness of the respiratory muscles leading to reduced loudness and pitch variability, which in turn results in strained voice and short phrases (prosody).

There are 12 pairs of cranial nerves. Of these 7 pairs of cranial nerves are most relevant for speech and hearing. The cranial nerves are already discussed in the section on *overview of speech production – speech subsystems*. The nuclei of these nerves are located in the pons or the medulla and they transmit sensory and/or motor impulses to and from the periphery and the CNS. Motor messages are sent from the CNS to the cranial nerve nuclei, and then to the musculature of the speech mechanism and other portions of the head, neck, shoulders, and the abdominal and thoracic viscera. Sensory messages emerge from the periphery and go to the cranial nerve nuclei and further to the thalamus. The thalamus, in turn, sends the messages to the sensory cortex. However, the only cranial nerve that does not follow this sensory route is the auditory nerve responsible for hearing and balance. Most of the cranial nerves have bilateral neural innervation, some have unilateral neural innervation, and some a mixture of bilateral and unilateral neural innervation from the corticobulbar tract of the CNS. Any unilateral lesion of a cranial nerve having bilateral neural innervation will result in less severe speech defects than that having unilateral neural innervation because the undamaged or the functional tract can compensate for the damaged one. In contrary, bilateral damage to bilateral tracts, and unilateral damage to unilateral tracts, will produce severe speech defects. Some examples are given below.

Bilateral damage to the sensory function and/or the motor function of *Trigeminal nerve* can affect articulation and prosody and reduced rate of speech. Unilateral damage to the motor function of the *Facial nerve* can result in mild articulation problems, and bilateral damage to the motor function can result in moderate to severe articulation problems, slow rate, and facial expression (pragmatics). Bilateral damage to the sensory function and/or the motor function of the *Trigeminal nerve* can result in articulation and slow rate of speech. Unilateral lesion of the *Vestibulocochlear nerve* that completely destroys the cochlea, auditory nerve, or cochlear nuclei may result in total deafness in that ear. Unilateral damage in the ascending auditory pathways and in the auditory cortex can lead to impaired hearing. Hearing problem can indirectly affect the speaker's loudness modulation, articulation, and prosody. Unilateral or bilateral damage in Heschl's gyrus can lead to auditory agnosia, where the individual has difficulty recognizing and identifying sounds in the environment, including speech. Unilateral damage to the motor function of the *Vagus nerve* can lead to problems in phonation - reduced pitch range, hoarseness, reduced loudness, short phrases, breathiness, dipsophobia -, resonance problems - mild hypernasality, nasal emission, and dysprosody - short phrases. Bilateral damage can affect phonation - short phrases, reduced loudness, breathiness, aphonia, inhalatory stridor, hoarseness, reduced pitch range, resonance - moderate to severe hypernasality, nasal emission -, articulation - weak pressure consonants, and prosody -short phrases, slow rate-. Bilateral damage to *Hypoglossal nerve* can cause mild to severe articulation problems, and reduced rate of speech.

4.2.19. The Neurosensory System

The neurosensory system is found in almost all the levels of the human nervous system. The important systems for speech and hearing are the sensory pathways of *general somatic functioning, the cranial nerves, vision and hearing, and the control circuits.* The *general somatic* (pain, touch, temperature, and proprioception) *sensory pathways* concerned with the limbs and the trunk make use of the spinal cord and spinal nerves. The *somatic sensory pathways* concerned with the head and speech mechanism make use of the cranial nerves. The sensory impulse from the peripheral organs passes through the spinal nerves through the dorsal portion of the cell body. Further from here, the sensory impulse passes through spinothalamic tracts to the thalamus, then to the internal capsule through thalamocortical tracts, and finally to the somatosensory area of the parietal lobe (postcentral gyrus). Sensory information about proprioception is required for speech as adjustments and compensations should take place under necessary circumstances. For example, speaking with food in mouth or speaking with prosthesis in the mouth.

The neurosensory system also contains special pathways used for vision and hearing. The *visual system*, with the help of the optic nerve, initiates with the eye's absorbing light from an image, sends the image through to the pupil. Following this, the image is inverted and reversed as it travels into the lens. The function of the lens is to focus and project the light onto the retina, which is a formation of nerve cells lining the inside of the eyeball. The visual impulse, with the help of the retina, reaches the optic nerve, and the optic chiasma. At this point, several of the fibers decussate and further move on to the lateral geniculate body of the thalamus, the primary center for vision and the visual association areas of the occipital lobe through the internal capsule. Lesions of the optic nerve and the primary visual cortex can lead to blindness. Lesions in the visual association cortex can lead to visual agnosia, alexia, and reading comprehension deficit. The *cochlear branch of the 8th cranial nerve* receives sensory impulses from the cochlea of the inner ear and transmits these impulses to the cochlear nuclear complex in the CNS. Most of the fibers decussate and travel to the superior olivary complex, and then to the medial geniculate body in the thalamus. The thalamus then sends the fibers to Heschl's gyrus, which is the primary hearing center in the temporal lobe of the cortex. Auditory and visual information is important for the production of speech and language. The auditory system is essential, and the visual system is also quite important, in the acquisition of speech and language. The auditory system helps maintain these throughout life. The sensory information received from the periphery is extremely important for the functioning of the basal ganglia and cerebellar *control circuits.*

4.2.20. The Autonomic Nervous System (ANS)

The autonomic nervous system (ANS) controls the involuntary activity of the body and is made up of a *sympathetic* and a *parasympathetic* division. The ANS is self-regulating and exists throughout the CNS and the PNS. The *sympathetic division* is responsible for activities such as speeding up the heart rate, constricting the peripheral blood vessels, raising blood pressure, raising the eyelids, redistributing blood, dilating the pupils, and decreasing contractions of the intestines. The sympathetic division creates internal adjustments and alerts the body to cope with stress and crises. In contrary, the *parasympathetic division* is responsible for slowing down the heart rate, increasing contractions of the intestines, increasing salivation, and increasing secretions of the glands in the gastro intestines. It is accountable for reducing internal activity and calming down the body. The ANS works all along with the endocrine system to sustain homeostasis and is controlled by the hypothalamus in the CNS. The ANS also has an indirect effect upon speech and language, such as the nervousness which may be felt before, during, or after certain speaking situations.

As previously described, the nervous system is responsible for several reflex movements such as respiratory activities, chewing etc. Some of these primary reflexes were modified to prelinguistic phonatory and articulatory patterns, and, then to skilled speech movements. That is, the reflexes of the respiratory system - breathing -, the laryngeal system – vocal fold reflexes –, articulatory system – chewing - is modified for speech which has evolved over a period of time, the path of which is not very clear till date.

4.3. Genetic Basis of Speech

The origin of speech has been a matter of study since long and has been attributed to divine origin, social pressure, echo, emotional outbursts, phonetic types, gesture, oral gesture, vocal play, social control, and social relation.

According to the *divine origin theory*, the origin of language is divine. According to Adam smith, the *social pressure theory*, the primitive man had to make his needs known to the other and started making some sounds to designate objects. In doing so some group of sounds were attached to certain objects and hence speech originated. The *bow wow theory* or the *Onomatopoetic* or *Echoic theory* put forth that objects were attached with names that resembled the sounds the objects produced. For example, the words *murmur, boom, snap, crash* etc. are echoic. However, it may not be true for all words. Miller criticized the echoic theory and traced a number of echoic words to their origin. For example, the word *thunder* was traced back to Indo-European root of the Sanskrit *tan* which means *to stretch*. Also, these echoes must have started after man started using speech and they are possible teaching by parents rather than imitation of sounds. According to the *interjectional theory*, the instance utterances under emotional strain or intense feeling are assigned by the listener to the emotions itself. Miller, following the analyses of language families, hypothesizes that speech was neither imitations nor interjections; but were phonetic types or basic modes of articulate utterances and names it as *phonetic type theory*. There are several other theories hypothesizing the origin of speech.

Results of studies on the course of speech development in a child indicate that, it generally does not follow exactly the same manner as the racial development. However, there are some similarities between the course of speech development and racial development. There is no inherent tendency or instinct to speak in neither the child nor the aboriginal man. Therefore, speech *may not be innate*. There exist a well-developed set of laryngeal and articulate utterances in both the child and the aboriginal man. The differences are that the aboriginal man had to create vocabulary and grammatical forms; but the child enters in to an environment in which these are already established. Since the child enters in to an environment in which vocabulary and grammatical forms already established, he gains mastery of language within the first few years of his life; but it must have taken several generations for the race to develop speech.

To learn speech, certain physiological and psychological factors are essential and in the absence of these, speech would be impossible. For example, a normal speech mechanism, normal nervous system, capacity for ideas are essential. An infant does not speak because either his physiological system is immature, or he does not have ideas. His activities are reflexive, involuntary in the beginning. The system becomes matured after several months or years. At birth, the child has sensory, neural, muscular and glandular structures. However, energy, in its various forms, called stimuli, impinges upon the sense organs which in turn generate neural impulses. As already described in the neural basis of speech, these impulses are conducted to various muscles due to which the human body works - digestion, vocalization, respiration and so on. At birth, all these responses are undifferentiated; the infant still performs natural biological functions. However, it is important to note that the child cries from the moment of birth.

We have already learnt that speech is an overlaid function and that the mechanisms used for speech had purely vegetative functions. Even after being used for speech the organs have not undergone any modifications. Most organs were biological but have undergone modifications in the course of time. The speech mechanism without undergoing modification has become biosocial. Such a development, most likely, can occur when the biosocial function involved had a significant survival value. Therefore, communication in human beings must have a significant survival value. The speech mechanism certainly develops and is anatomically and physiologically different at adulthood than what it was at birth. Thus, the mechanism involved in speech production together with the neuromuscular complexes, is not only a biological mechanism but is also a biosocial mechanism.

The first linguistic experience of the infant consists not in expression by speech or gesture, but in the understanding of language (Revesz, 1953). The infant responds to the human voice at an early age. But whether it is innate

Bases of Speech and Language 137

or through conditioned learning is not known. Speech development has already been explained in earlier section. It consists of birth cry, babbling, reduplicated babbling/ lalling, first word and so on.

However, it is unknown as to how language evolved in humans. It might reside in genes - either new genes, or changes in old genes that gives them new functions. Genes carry hereditary biological information that determines much about who we are, from our hair color to our height to which hand we use to write with. Research on the genetic basis of speech suggests one particular gene, called FOXP2, one of the few genes that have been associated with the capacity for human speech and language. "FOXP2 works in an interesting way in that it turns other things on and off and regulates other genes. In a cell, FOXP2 acts like a master switch, producing a protein that binds to other genes and increases or decreases their activity" (Konopka and colleagues, 2009).

Human FOXP2 protein is almost identical to the version found in our closest primate relative, the chimpanzee. FOXP2 protein is made up of hundreds of amino acids of which just two amino acids are different between human and chimpanzee (Geschwind, 2009). "Results of studies by other researchers have suggested that the amino acid composition of the human FOXP2 protein might have changed at about the same time in evolutionary history that humans started to speak. It has been reported that the human and chimpanzee versions of FOXP2 function differently in human brain cells, targeting different genes and triggering different levels of gene activity" (Konopka and colleagues, 2009).

Many of the genes and proteins affected by FOXP2 are known to have functions in the brain. However, others may be involved in the development of the physical apparatus of speech, like the larynx and vocal folds as a change in vocal anatomy and in the brain is essential to have spoken language. Speech and language are connected, and at least one connection may be via FOXP2 (Geschwind, 2009).

Conclusion

This chapter covered bases of speech and language. An overview of speech production along with speech sub-systems active in speech production such as the nervous system, respiratory system, laryngeal system, and resonatory/articulatory system along with figures and illustrations were provided. The concept of sound, how it is generated, periodic and aperiodic sounds, and concepts such as cycle, displacement, period, frequency, amplitude related to sound were covered. Simple harmonic motion, sine wave, complex wave, and physical properties of the vibrating system such as elasticity, inertia, damping, and propagation of sound waves including transverse and longitudinal waves were included. Further other properties of sound such as absorption, reflection of sound, free and forced vibration and resonance were covered. Following this and having learnt about sound in detail, the chapter covered how the speech mechanism can be a sound generator. To make the concept clear, properties of the vocal tract, and how speech can be considered as an acoustic wave were included. Further, the Acoustic theory of speech production, the source of speech – Noise, voice, Noise + voice -, and filter characteristics of the vocal tract with illustrations were provided. The social basis of speech was dealt in brief, and under the neurological basis of speech, the concepts of the Neuron, nerve excitation, conduction of nerve impulse, and neurotransmitters such as Acetylcholine, Monoamines, Norepinephrine, Serotonin, & GABA or γ-aminobutyric acid were covered. The human nervous system, including the Brain, cerebral Hemispheres, cerebellum, brainstem, spinal Cord, meninges, ventricles, Blood Supply to the nervous system, motor System for Speech, upper and lower motor neurons, peripheral Nervous System, neurosensory System, and autonomic nervous system. The genetic basis of speech covered divine origin theory, social pressure theory, the bow wow theory or the Onomatopoetic or Echoic theory. In brief the chapter sufficiently covered bases of speech.

REFERENCES

ANSI S1.1-1994 Retrieved from https://infostore.saiglobal.com/en-au/standards/ansi-s1-1-1994-799670/. Accessed March 15.

ANSI S1.1-1994. *American National Standard: Acoustic Terminology. Sec 3.03*. Accessed March 15.

ANSI/ASA S1.1-2013 Retrieved from https://en.wikipedia.org/wiki/ANSI/ASA_S1.1-2013 Accessed March 15.

Cooley, C. H. 1909. *Primary Groups*. New York: Charles Scribner's Sons.

Damasio, A. 1994. *Descartes' error*. New York: G.P. Putnam's Sons.

Duffy, J. R. 2005. *Motor speech disorders: Substrates, differential diagnosis and management*. St. Louis: Mosby/Elsevier.

Fant, G. 1960. *Acoustic theory of speech production*. Mouton: The Hague.

Fry, D. B. 1979. *The Physics of Speech*. Cambridge: Cambridge University Press.

Garey L. J. 2006. *Brodmann's Localisation in the Cerebral Cortex*. New York: Springer. ISBN 978-0387-26917-7.

Geschwind, D. H. 2009. Cited in Konopka, G., Bomar, J. M., Winden, K, Coppola, G., Jonsson, Z. O., Gao, F., Peng, S, Preuss, T., Wohlschlege, J. A., and Geschwind, D. H. 2009. "Human-specific transcriptional regulation of CNS development genes by FOXP2." *Nature*, Vol. 462|12.

Gray, G. W., and Wise, C. M. 1959. *The Basis of Speech*. New York: Harper & Row.

Henry Pieron, 1956. "Geza Revesz: 1878-1955." *The American Journal of Psychology*, Vol. 69, No. 1. 139-141.

Herries, J. (1974). *The elements of speech*. London: Scholar Press.

http://en.wikipedia.org/wiki/Resonance. Accessed March 2.

Kent, R. D., and Read, C. 1995. *The acoustic analysis of speech*. London: Whurr Publishers.

Konopka, G., Bomar, J. M., Winden, K., Coppola, G., Jonsson, Z. O., Gao, F., Peng, S., Preuss, T. M., Wohlschlegel, J. A., and Geschwind, D. H. 2009. "Human-specific transcriptional regulation of CNS development genes by FOXP2." *Nature*, 462, 213-217.

Ladefoged, P. 1962. *Elements of Acoustic Phonetics*, Chicago: University of Chicago Press.

Mahabharata (Ve:davya:sa, Dwapara yuga). 1967. Edited by T. R. Krishnacharya & T. R. Vyasacarya Nirnayasagara Press. Bombay. 12-320-91 to 92.

Meyer-Eppler, W. 1953. "Zum Erzeugungsmechanismus des Gerauschlaute." *Z. fiir Phonetik* 314, 196-212.

News & Comment Memorial. 1880. "Dr. Paul Broca." *Science*. 1 (9): 93. 21 August 1880. doi:10.1126/science.os-1.9.93. JSTOR 2900242. Accessed March 17.

Raphael, L. J., Bordon, G. J., & Harris, K. S. (2006). *Speech Science Primer: Physiology, Acoustics, and Perception of Speech*. (6th Ed.). Lippincott: Williams and Wilkins.

Schroeder, J. 2000. "Nagarjuna. Upa:ya kausalya hr.daya." *Phylosophy East and West*. Vol. 50, 4.

Speaks, C. E. 2005. *Introduction to Sound: Acoustics for the Hearing and Speech Sciences* (3rd Edition). Canada: Nelson Education Ltd.

Sreedevi, N. 2015. Personal Communication.

Travis, L. E. 1971. *Handbook of Speech Pathology and Audiology*. New York: Aplleton-Century Crofts. 0390885398 (ISBN13: 9780390885395).

Walters, E. G. 1969. *Fundamentals of Telephone Communication Systems*. New York: Western Electric Company. p. 2.1.

Wernicke, C. 1848 – 1905. Retrieved from https://en.wikipedia.org/wiki/Carl_Wernicke. Accessed February 25.

Chapter 3

SOUND INTENSITY AND CONCEPT OF DECIBEL

INTRODUCTION

Having learnt about sound in detail in the previous chapter, it is important to learn about some basic concepts such as sound energy, sound power, sound pressure, sound intensity level, and decibel in order to understand the human hearing mechanism. In this chapter, we shall learn about some of these concepts. *Sound energy* is one of the forms of energy, and *sound power* is the rate at which sound energy is emitted, reflected, transmitted or received, per unit time. The human ear is capable of hearing sound powers that range from 10^{-12} W to 10-100 W. *Sound power level* is the expression of sound power relative to the threshold of hearing in a logarithmic scale. *Sound intensity* is the power carried by sound waves per unit area. *Sound power* is equal to the area multiplied by sound intensity. *Sound pressure* is the local pressure deviation from the ambient atmospheric pressure, caused by a sound wave. Hence it is the difference between the pressure produced by a sound wave and the ambient pressure of the medium it is passing through, and is a product of sound intensity and sound particle velocity. Human hearing is directly sensitive to sound pressure. *Sound intensity level* is the level of the intensity of a sound relative to a reference value. The concepts of sound pressure, intensity, and power are most often confused. Sound pressure can be measured directly. Sound intensity and power are related to pressure and are distinct from sound pressure. The *decibel* (dB) is used to measure sound level. The *decibel* (dB) is a logarithmic unit used to express the ratio of one value of a physical property to another. Hence, when the level of a sound is represented in decibel, a reference is essential. A zero dB occurs when the intensity of the sound in question is equal to the reference level. The human ear is capable of hearing a very large range of sounds. The ratio is more than a million. To deal with such a range, *logarithmic units* are useful. The log of a million is 6, and hence this ratio represents a difference of 120 dB. Logarithmic measures are also useful when a sound increases or decreases exponentially over time. Hence *decibel* is used as a unit to express sound intensity.

1. ACOUSTIC ENERGY AND POWER, ABSOLUTE AND RELATIVE UNITS – IMPORTANCE OF REFERENCE

1.1. Acoustic Power or Sound Power

Acoustic power or Sound power "is the rate at which sound energy is emitted, reflected, transmitted or received, per unit time" (Baken, & Orlikoff, 2000*)*. The unit of sound power is the watt (W). It is the power of the sound force on a surface of the medium of propagation of the sound wave. Acoustic power is neither room-dependent nor distance-dependent. Sound power of a source is the total power emitted by that source in all directions, while the sound pressure is a measurement at a point in space near the source.

Sound power, denoted as P, is defined by

$$P = f^*v = Apu * v = Apv \tag{7}$$

where, f is the sound force of unit vector u, v is the particle velocity of projection v along u, A is the area, p is the sound pressure (Landau & Lifchitz, 1987)

In a medium, the sound power is given by

$$P = \frac{Ap^2}{\rho c} \cos \theta,$$

(8)

where, A is the area of the surface, ρ is the mass density, c is the sound velocity, θ is the angle between the direction of propagation of the sound and the normal to the surface.

For example, if the sound at sound pressure level (SPL) is 85 dB or p = 0.356 or ρ = 1.2 kg·m^{-3} Pa in air, c = 343 m·s^{-1}) through a surface of area A = 1 m^2 normal to the direction of propagation, and $\theta = 0\,°$ (cos 0 ° = 1), then sound energy $P = [1^{2*} (1.2)^2 / (1.2^* 343)]\, 1 = 0.3$ mW.

1.2. Sound Power Level

Sound power level is the expression of sound power relative to the threshold of hearing (10^{-12} W) in a logarithmic decibel scale as follows:

$$L_N = 10 \log (N/N_{ref})$$

(9)

where, L_N is the sound power level, N is sound power in Watts, N_{ref} is 10^{-12}, that is the reference sound power.

For example, if the sound power is 0.0015 W, the sound power level can be calculated as

$$L_N = 10 \log (N/N_{ref})$$

(10)

$$L_N = 10 \log (0.0015\ W/\ 10^{-12}\ W) = 91.8\ dB$$

(11)

144   *S. R. Savithri*

Table 5 shows examples of sound power in Watts and sound power level in decibels from some sources.

Table 5. Examples of sound power in Watts and sound power level in decibels from some sources

Situation and sound source	Sound power (W)	Sound power level (dB ref 10^{-12} W)
Saturn V rocket	100,000,000	200
Turbojet engine	100,000	170
Turbofan aircraft at take-off	1,000	150
Machine gun Large pipe organ	10	130
Symphony orchestra Heavy thunder Sonic boom	1	120
Rock concert Chain saw Accelerating motorcycle	0.1	110
Lawn mower Car at highway speed Subway steel wheels	0.01	10
Large diesel vehicle	0.001	90
Loud alarm clock	0.0001	80
Relatively quiet vacuum cleaner	10^{-5}	70
Hair dryer	10^{-6}	60
Radio or TV	10^{-7}	50
Refrigerator Low voice	10^{-8}	40
Quiet conversation	10^{-9}	30
Whisper of one person Wristwatch ticking	10^{-10}	20
Human breath of one person	10^{-11}	10
Reference value	10^{-12}	0

The human ear is capable of hearing sound powers that range from 10^{-12} W to 10-100 W, which is a range of $10/ 10^{-12} = 10^{13}$.

Acoustic power or sound power is related to sound intensity as follows:

$$P = AI, \tag{12}$$

where, A is the area and I is the sound intensity

Sound Intensity and Concept of Decibel 145

Sound power is also related sound energy density:

P = Acw, (13)

Where, c is the speed of sound, w is the sound energy density.

1.3. Sound Intensity and Intensity Levels –Absolute and Relative Measurements

Sound intensity or acoustic intensity is defined as the power carried by sound waves per unit area. The SI unit of sound intensity is watt per square meter (W/m^2) (retrieved from https://en.wikipedia.org/wiki/Sound_intensity). Sound intensity is not the same physical quantity as sound pressure. However, sound intensity and sound pressure are related. Hearing is directly sensitive to sound pressure.

Sound intensity, denoted I, is defined by

I = pv, where p is the sound pressure and v is the particle velocity.

Both I and v are vectors, that is, both have a direction as well as a magnitude. The direction of sound intensity is the average direction in which energy is flowing. The average sound intensity during time T is given by

$$\langle \mathbf{I} \rangle = \frac{1}{T} \int_0^T p(t)\mathbf{v}(t)\, dt.$$ (14)

Intensity of Sound $= 2\pi^2 n^2 A^2 \rho v$ (15)

where, n is frequency of sound, A is the Amplitude of sound wave, v is velocity of sound, and ρ is density of medium in which sound is travelling.

1.3.1. Sound Intensity and Intensity Levels –Absolute and Relative Measurements

Sound intensity level (SIL) or acoustic intensity level is the level of the intensity of a sound relative to a reference value expressed in a logarithmic quantity. It is denoted by L_I, expressed in dB, and defined as follows:

$$L_I = \frac{1}{2} \ln \left(\frac{I}{I_0} \right) \text{Np} = \log_{10} \left(\frac{I}{I_0} \right) \text{B} = 10 \log_{10} \left(\frac{I}{I_0} \right) \text{dB},$$

(16)

where, I is the sound intensity, I_0 is the reference sound intensity, 1 Np = 1 is the neper, 1 B = (1/2) ln (10) is the bel, 1 dB = (1/20), ln (10) is the decibel.

The commonly used reference sound intensity in air is (Roeser, Valente, & Hosford-Dunn, 2007)

$$I_0 = 1 \text{ pW/m}^2$$

(17)

The reference sound intensity I_0 is defined such that a progressive plane wave has the same value of sound intensity level (SIL) and sound pressure level (SPL) as

$$I \, \alpha \, p^2$$

(18)

SIL will be equal to SPL when

$$\frac{I}{I_0} = \frac{p^2}{p_0^2},$$

(19)

where, $P_0 = 20 \, \mu$Pa, which is the reference sound pressure level.

2. Bel and Decibels, Sound Pressure and Decibel Sound Pressure Levels, Relationship between Intensity and Pressure

The definition of the decibel is based on the measurement of power in telephony of the early 20th century in the Bell System in the United States. One decibel is one tenth (deci) of one bel, named in honor of Alexander Graham Bell. The *decibel* (dB) is a logarithmic unit used to express the ratio of one value of a physical property to another, and may be used to express a change in value (e.g., +1 dB or -1 dB) or an absolute value. In the latter case, it expresses the ratio of a value to a reference value; when used in this way, the decibel symbol should be appended with a suffix that indicates the reference value or some other property. For example, if the reference value is 1 volt, then the suffix is "V," i.e., "20 dBV," and if the reference value is one milliwatt, then the suffix is "m," i.e., "20 dBm" (retrieved from http://www.analog.com/en/design-center/interactive-design-tools/ dbconvert.html). However, sound pressure level is referenced to the "threshold of hearing" (generally given as 20 micropascals at 1 kHz), and the suffix is "SPL" (i.e., "60 dB SPL") (retrieved from http://www.aes.org/par/s/#SPL)

Two different scales are used to express a ratio in decibels depending on the nature of the quantities- *field quantity* ratio or *power quantity* ratio -. Field quantity ratio is also named as *root-power* ratio or *amplitude* ratio. In power quantities expressions, the number of decibels is ten times the logarithm to base 10 of the ratio of two power quantities (*IEEE Standard, 2000*). It means that a change in power by a factor of 10 corresponds to a 10 dB change in level. However, in expressing field quantities, a change in amplitude by a factor of 10 corresponds to a 20 dB change in level. This extra factor of two is due to the logarithm of the quadratic relationship between power and amplitude. The decibel scales differ so that direct comparisons can be made between related power and field quantities when they are expressed in decibels.

148   *S. R. Savithri*

In the International System of Quantities, the decibel is defined as a unit of measurement for quantities of type level or level difference, which are defined as the logarithm of the ratio of power- or field-type quantities.

2.1. Sound Pressure or Acoustic Pressure

Sound pressure or acoustic pressure is the local pressure deviation from the ambient (average, or equilibrium) atmospheric pressure, caused by a sound wave. Hence it is the difference between the pressure produced by a sound wave and the ambient pressure of the medium it is passing through. In air, sound pressure can be measured using a microphone, and in water with a hydrophone. The unit of sound pressure is the pascal (Pa).

The lowest sound pressure possible to hear is approximately *2 10^{-5} Pa (20 micro Pascal, 0.02 mPa) or 2 ten billionths* of an atmosphere. The minimum audible level occurs between *3000 and 4000 Hz*. For a normal human ear pain is experienced at sound pressures of order *60 Pa* or 6 10^{-4} atmospheres.

2.2. Sound Pressure Level (Decibels)

It is convenient to express sound pressure with the logarithmic decibel scale related to the lowest human audible sound, that is *2 10^{-5} Pa or 0 dB*.

Sound Pressure Level can be expressed as:

$$L_p = 10 \log (p^2 / p_{ref}^2) \qquad\qquad (20)$$
$$= 10 \log (p / p_{ref})^2$$
$$= 20 \log (p / p_{ref})$$

where,

$$L_p = sound\ pressure\ level\ (dB)$$
$$p = sound\ pressure\ (Pa)$$

$p_{ref} = 2 \ 10^{-5}$ *[reference sound pressure (Pa])*

A doubling of sound pressure results in increase of sound pressure level by *6 dB or 20 log (2).*

2.3. Sound Intensity

Sound Intensity is the rate of energy flow across a unit area (power per unit area) or it is the product of sound pressure and sound particle velocity. The concepts of sound pressure, intensity, and power are easily confused. Sound pressure can be measured directly. Sound intensity and power are related to pressure but have important distinctions. Sound intensity level (Nave, 2006) can be measures as

Sound Intensity Level (IL) – 10 log (I/I_0),
where $I_0 = 10^{-12}$ watts/meter^2 (21)

In a free field, intensity varies as $1/r^2$ for an omni-directional source. This corresponds to a 6 dB decrease in intensity for each doubling of distance from the source. Further, in a free field, IL and SPL are nearly equal for a single source. Two equal sources produce a 3 dB increase in sound power level. Two equal sources produce a 3 dB increase in sound pressure level, assuming no interference. Two 80 dB sources add to produce an 83 dB SPL.

3. CHARACTERISTICS AND APPLICATION OF DECIBELS

The *decibel* (dB) is used to measure sound level. It is also widely used in electronics, signals and communication. It is a *logarithmic way of describing a ratio.* The ratio may be power, sound pressure, voltage or intensity or several other things. It is expressed in a logarithmic scale. One decibel is close to the Just Noticeable Difference (JND) for sound level.

150   *S. R. Savithri*

Let us revise logarithm. Suppose we write 10^2. It means $10*10 = 100$; $10^4 = 10*10*10*10 = 10,000$. Here the exponent 2 or 4 tells us how many times to multiply the base (10 in this example) by itself. In this example, 2 is the log of 100 and 4 is the log of 10000. So 10^1 means that there is only one 10 in the product, so 1 is the log of 10, or in other words $10^1 = 10$. The factor 10 in the definition puts the 'deci' in decibel.

We can also have negative logarithms. 10^{-2} means 0.01, which is 1/100; $10^{-n} = 1/10^n$ and so on. Suppose we have $(10^2)^3$. Let us first derive $10^2 = 100$. So, $100^3 = 100*100*100 = 1,000,000 = 10^6$. Here exponents 2 and 3 are whole numbers. However, they need not be whole numbers

The definition of the logarithm of a number a (to base 10) is $10^{\log a} = a$. In other words, the log of the number a is the power to which you must raise 10 to get the number a. For example, $3.1623^2 = 10$ can be written as $3.1623^2 = (10^{\log 3.1623})^2 = 10 = 10^1$.

Having revised logarithm, suppose we have two loudspeakers, the first playing a sound with power P_1, and another playing a louder version of the same sound with power P_2, but everything else (distance, frequency) is kept the same. The difference in decibels between the two speakers can be defined to be

$$10 \log (P_2/P_1) \text{ dB, where the log is to base 10.} \tag{22}$$

If the second speaker produces twice as much power than the first, the difference in dB is

$$10 \log (P_2/P_1) = 10 \log 2 = 3 \text{ dB.} \tag{23}$$

If the second speaker had 10 times the power of the first, the difference in dB would be

$$10 \log (P_2/P_1) = 10 \log 10 = 10 \text{ dB.} \tag{24}$$

If the second speaker had ten lakhs times the power of the first, the difference in dB would be

Sound Intensity and Concept of Decibel   151

$$10 \log (P_2/P_1) = 10 \log 1,000,000 = 60 \text{ dB.} \qquad (25)$$

The above example shows that decibel scales can describe very big ratios using numbers of small size. But remember that the decibel describes a *ratio*. Till now we learnt only the ratio of powers, but not the power either of the speakers radiates.

Sound is usually measured with microphones and they respond approximately proportionally to the sound pressure, p. The power in a sound wave, all else being equal, is the square of the pressure. In the same way, electrical power in a resistor is the square of the voltage. The log of the square of x is just 2 log x, so this introduces a *factor of 2* when we convert to decibels for pressures. The difference in sound pressure level between two sounds with p_1 and p_2 is therefore:

$$20 \log (p_2/p_1) \text{ dB} = 10 \log (p_2^2/p_1^2) \text{ dB} = 10 \log (P_2/P_1) \text{ dB,} \qquad (26)$$

Where, the log is to base 10

Suppose you halve the sound power, then the log of 2 is 0.3. So the log of 1/2 is - 0.3. Thus, if you halve the power, you reduce the power and the sound level by 3 dB. If you halve it again to 1/4 of the original power, you are reducing the level by another 3 dB. If you keep on halving the power, the following will be the ratios.

P,	$\frac{p}{\sqrt{2}}$,	$\frac{p}{2}$,	$\frac{p}{2\sqrt{2}}$,	$\frac{p}{4}$,	$\frac{p}{4\sqrt{2}}$,	$\frac{p}{8}$,	$\frac{p}{8\sqrt{2}}$,
I,	$\frac{I}{2}$,	$\frac{I}{4}$,	$\frac{I}{8}$,	$\frac{I}{16}$,	$\frac{I}{32}$,	$\frac{I}{64}$,	$\frac{I}{128}$,
L,	L–3dB,	L–6dB,	L–9dB,	L–12dB,	L–15dB,	L–18dB,	L–21dB

If we add two identical sounds, is the intensity doubled (increase in 3 dB) or the pressure doubled? (Increase of 6 dB)? This is a frequently asked question, and it is a little subtle.

S. R. Savithri

Assume that you have a completely linear amplifier and speaker. If the input is the same signal to both amplifiers, each amplifier will produce the same amount of electrical power, so the output sound power is only doubled. That is, the intensity in the sound field is doubled. If your ear is equidistant from the two speakers, then the two pressure waves will add in phase resulting in double the sound pressure at the ear. Hence, you will hear a level 6 dB higher when the second amplifier is turned on. Thus, if you double the voltage at the input, you will double the sound pressure it gives out, which produces four times as much energy, four times as much intensity everywhere in the sound field, and thus a uniform increase in sound level of 6 dB. However, if you are half a wavelength far away from one speaker than from the other, then two pressure waves will add one half cycle out of phase and the sound pressure will be zero. So, the sound intensity is four times as great in some places, zero in others, and intermediate values in most places. Integrating this over all space, the *total* power will be doubled. For example, if two signals have pressure amplitude p_m and a phase difference θ, then their sum would be equal to $2p_m(1+\cos\theta)$. The power is proportional to the amplitude squared, and so proportional to $4p_m^2(1+\cos\theta)^2$. The average of $(1+\cos\theta)^2$ over all θ is ½. Hence, the average of the whole term over all possible phase differences is $2p_m^2$. So again, on average doubling the power results in an increase of 3 dB in sound level. Usually sound levels are given in whole numbers and not in decimal places because sound levels differing by less than 1 dB are hard to distinguish.

We have already learnt that decibel is a ratio. Hence, when the level of a sound is represented in decibel, a reference is essential. For SPL, the reference level is 20 micro pascals (20 μPa), or 0.02 mPa, which is very low (Two ten billionths of an atmosphere). However, it is the limit of sensitivity of the human ear. For example, an SPL of 86 dB means $20 \log (p_2/p_1) = 86$ dB, where p_1 is the sound pressure of the reference level, and p_2 that of the sound in question and divide both sides by 20. That is, $\log (p_2/p_1) = 4.3$ or $p_2/p_1 = 10^{4.3}$. Here 4 is the log of 10,000, 0. 3 is the log of 2, so this sound has a pressure 20 thousand times greater than that of the reference level ($p_2/p_1 = 20,000$). 86 dB is a loud sound; however, it is not a dangerous level

Sound Intensity and Concept of Decibel 153

of sound, if it is not maintained for very long. Table 6 shows the intensity and the corresponding dB levels.

Table 6. Intensity and the corresponding dB levels

Intensity	-----	dB
$1Wm^{-2}$	-----	120
$1mWm^{-2}$	-----	90
$1\mu Wm^{-2}$	-----	60
$1nWm^{-2}$	-----	30
$1pWm^{-2}$	-----	0

A zero dB occurs when the intensity of the sound in question is equal to the reference level. i.e., it is the sound level corresponding to 0.02 mPa. In such a case, sound level $= 20 \log (p_{measured}/p_{reference}) = 20 \log 1 = 0$ dB. Recalling that the dB measure is a ratio, 0 dB does not mean no sound; on the other hand, it means the level of the sound is equal to that of the reference level. It is a small pressure but not zero. It is possible to have negative sound pressure. For example, -20 dB means that the sound in question has a pressure 10 times smaller than that of the reference pressure, i.e., 2 μPa or 0.02 mPa.

Not all sound pressures are equally loud because the human ear does not respond equally to all frequencies. The human ear is more sensitive to sounds in the frequency range about 1 kHz to 4 kHz than to very low or high frequency sounds. The human ear is capable of hearing a very large range of sounds. The ratio is more than a million. To deal with such a range, *logarithmic units* are useful. The log of a million is 6, and hence this ratio represents a difference of 120 dB. Logarithmic measures are also useful when a sound increases or decreases exponentially over time. This happens in many applications involving proportional gain or proportional loss. *Hence decibel is used.*

CONCLUSION

The previous chapter covered sound and its properties, transmission of sound and speech as a sound. In this chapter, the basic concepts of sound related to hearing were covered. The chapter included the definitions of sound energy, and sound power. It also included the sound powers that the human ear is capable of hearing. Further, the definitions of sound power level, sound intensity, and the relation between sound power and sound intensity were covered. Meaning of sound pressure and its relation with sound intensity were incorporated. The sensitivity of human hearing with sound pressure, definition of sound intensity level, and the relation of sound pressure to sound intensity and power were discussed. The concept of decibel (dB) to measure sound level was introduced and the reason for the use of dB as a unit to express sound intensity was covered. These concepts and the chapter as a whole will serve as a firm basis for the understanding of human hearing mechanism.

REFERENCES

Baken, R. J., and Orlikoff, R. F. 2000. *Clinical Measurement of Speech and Voice.* (2nd Ed.). San Diago: Singular Publishing Co.

Fries, B., and Fries, M. 2005. *Digital Audio Essentials.* California: O'Reilly Media. p. 147.

http://www.aes.org/par/s/#SPL. Accessed February 8.

https://en.wikipedia.org/wiki/Sound_intensity. Accessed February 8.

IEEE Standard 100 Dictionary of IEEE Standards Terms, 2000. Seventh Edition, New York: The Institute of Electrical and Electronics Engineering, 288.

Landau, L. D., and Lifchitz, E. M. 1987. *Course of Theoretical Physics, Vol. 6: Fluid Mechanics* (2nd Ed.). Oxford: Pergamon Press.

"Letter symbols to be used in electrical technology – Part 3: Logarithmic and related quantities, and their units." 2002. *IEC 60027-3 Ed. 3.0,*

International Electrotechnical Commission, 19 July 2002. Accessed February 8.

Roeser, R., Valente, M. V., and Hosford-Dunn, H. (2007). *Audiology: Diagnosis*. New York: Thieme Publishers.

Chapter 4

AUDIBILITY AND HEARING

INTRODUCTION

This chapter covers hearing mechanism & the basic concepts related to hearing and its measurements. The ear is the sensory organ that is responsible for hearing and the maintenance of equilibrium, by detecting the body position and of head movement. It has three parts: the outer, middle, and inner ear. The outer or external ear is visible and is outside the skull; but the middle and the inner ear are inside the temporal bone. The external ear is made up of pinna, the external auditory canal, and the tympanic membrane. The middle ear consists of the tympanic cavity, an air-filled cavity, 3 small bones or ossicles - Malleus, Incus, & Stapes, the smallest bone in the body -, and 2 skeletal muscles - the tensor tympani attached to the malleus and the stapedius attached to the stapes. The tympanic cavity is an air-filled cavity. The outer wall of the cavity forms the tympanic membrane or eardrum, which communicates proximally with the nasopharynx by the Eustachian tubes. The Eustachian tubes maintain pressure equilibrium in the tympanic cavity with that on the outside. The middle ear and the inner ear are connected by two small openings – oval window, round window - closed by the membranes. The foot plate of the Stapes covers the oval window. A flexible secondary tympanic membrane covers the round window and the round window is responsible for equalizing the pressure on either side of the tympanic membrane. The inner ear contains the sensory apparatus and consists of a bony shell, the bony labyrinth which has two parts. The anterior part is the cochlea which is the actual organ of hearing. The posterior part of the bony labyrinth has the vestibule and the semi-circular canals, which are responsible for equilibrium. The organ of Corti, situated in the cochlear canal, has inner (around 3500) and outer hair cells (around 11,500) and is responsible for the transduction of acoustic stimuli. All the auditory information is transduced by these 15,000 hair cells. Of the hair cells, the inner hair cells are of vital importance, as they form synapses with approximately 90% of the 30,000 primary auditory neurons. The bodies of the cochlear sensory cells in the basilar membrane are surrounded by nerve terminals, and their axons (approximately 30,000 in number) form the cochlear nerve. The cochlear nerve crosses the inner ear canal and transcends to the central structures of the brain stem. The auditory fibers enter the temporal lobe, the part of the cerebral cortex that is responsible for the perception. The basic function of the ear is hearing. Sound waves passing through the external auditory canal hit the tympanic membrane, which in turn vibrates. This vibration is transmitted to the Malleus, Incus and Stapes. Also, the middle ear has a resonance frequency between 1000 to 2000 Hz. When the foot of the stapes moves, it causes waves to form in the liquid within the vestibular canal. The speed of sound waves propagating through the ear depends on the elasticity of the basilar membrane. The inner hair cells, the mechanoreceptors, transform the acoustic signals into electric messages and send it to the central nervous system.

The human ear can perceive frequencies between 16 Hz-25,000 Hz, sound pressures between 20 µPa to 20 Pa. The frequency-discrimination threshold or the minimal detectable difference in frequency is 1.5 Hz up to 500 Hz, and 0.3% of the stimulus frequency at higher frequencies. The minimum audible level or absolute threshold of hearing or auditory threshold is the minimum sound level of a pure tone that an average human ear with normal hearing can hear when no other sound is present.

The chapter further covers procedures for estimation of audible levels that include the method of limits, the method of constant stimuli, and the method of adjustment with Forced-choice method, Adaptive methods, Staircase' methods or up-down methods and Bekesy's tracking method. Further, for a better understanding of hearing concepts of Minimum audible pressure and field, Missing six dB and related issues are introduced. Minimum audible pressure or MAP is the minimum level of a tone which can be presented via headphones to a participant at the minimum threshold of audibility. Minimum audible field is the threshold before which a tone cannot be heard by a participant. Auditory threshold refers to the minimum level of sound that can be detected and reported by an organism. There are other scales to measure loudness namely phon and sone. The phon is a unit of loudness level for pure tones and the sone, is also a unit of loudness and the sone scale is linear. Also, the Audiometric zero, Reference equivalent threshold sound pressure levels and hearing levels, Sensation levels, Threshold of pain, Most comfortable levels, Uncomfortable Listening Level (UCL), and Acceptable Noise Level (ANL) are discussed.

1. HEARING RANGE – INTENSITY AND FREQUENCY

1.1. Hearing Mechanism

Before going on to the hearing range, we shall learn about the hearing mechanism in brief. The ear is the sensory organ that is responsible for hearing and the maintenance of equilibrium, by detecting the body position and of head movement. It has three parts: the outer, middle, and inner ear. The outer or external ear is visible and is outside the skull; but the middle and the inner ear are inside the temporal bone.

The external ear is made up of pinna, the external auditory canal, and the tympanic membrane. The *pinna* is a projecting elastic cartilage covered with skin. The most prominent outer ridge of the pinna is the helix and the lobule is the soft flexible part. The lower part of the lobule is made up of fibrous and adipose tissue and is richly supplied with blood capillaries. The functioning of pinna is to sense sounds and collect it. The *external auditory canal* is a tubular passage, an irregularly-shaped cylinder approximately 25 mm long which is lined by glands secreting wax. The exterior part of the external auditory canal is supported by cartilage and the interior part is supported by bone. The external auditory canal is internally lined by stratified epithelium or hairy skin, and ceruminous glands. The ceruminous glands are adapted sweat glands that secrete the cerumen which is a waxy substance. The ear wax prevents the foreign bodies entering the ear. The *tympanic membrane* separates the tympanic cavity from the external auditory meatus. It is a thin and semi-transparent, and oval membrane. However, it is to some extent broader on top than below. The central part of the tympanic membrane is called the umbo. The handle of the malleus, which is one of the small bones of the middle ear, is tightly attached to the internal surface of the tympanic membrane. The external ear directs sound waves towards the tympanic membrane. The sound waves in turn produce pressure changes on the surface of the tympanic membrane or vibration of the tympanic membrane. Thus, the tympanic membrane acts as a resonator that reproduces the vibration of sound. Figure 83 shows the parts of human ear.

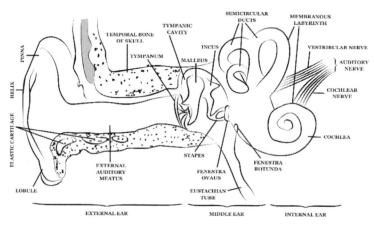

Source: http://www.biologydiscussion.com/human-body/ear/human-ear-structure-and-functions-with-diagram/47558.

Figure 83. Parts of human ear.

The middle ear consists of the tympanic cavity, 3 small bones or ossicles, and 2 skeletal muscles. The *tympanic cavity* is an air-filled cavity. The outer wall of the cavity forms the tympanic membrane or eardrum, which communicates proximally with the nasopharynx by the Eustachian tubes. The Eustachian tubes maintain pressure equilibrium in the tympanic cavity with that on the outside. If one tries to swallow, the pressure equalization happens, and the temporary loss of hearing, caused by rapid change in pressure as in case of fast elevators, landing airplanes, will be regained. The tympanic cavity carries the extra sound to the pharynx through Eustachian tube. The middle ear also has a small flexible chain of three small bones or *ear ossicles*. These are termed the *Malleus*, which is hammer shaped, the *Incus*, which is anvil shaped, and the *Stapes*, that is stirrup shaped. The Malleus is attached to the tympanic membrane on the outer side and to the incus on the inner side. The Incus is attached to the stapes, and the Stapes in turn is attached to the oval membrane that covers the fenestra ovalis or oval window of the inner ear. Of the three ossicles, Malleus is the largest and Stapes is smallest. Stapes is also the smallest bone in the body. The ossicles convert the acoustic energy to mechanical energy and transmit sound waves from external to the internal ear. The ossicles help in increasing the intensity of sound waves by about twenty times. Two skeletal muscles, the *tensor tympani* attached to the malleus and the *stapedius* attached to the stapes, are also present in the middle ear. Stapedius is the smallest muscle in the body. The middle ear and the inner ear are connected by two small openings closed by the membranes. These openings are fenestra ovalis or *oval window*, and fenestra rotunda or *round window*. The foot plate of the Stapes covers the oval window. A flexible secondary tympanic membrane covers the round window and the round window is responsible for equalizing the pressure on either side of the tympanic membrane.

The *inner ear* contains the sensory apparatus and consists of a bony shell, the bony labyrinth. The bony labyrinth has two parts. The anterior part is the *cochlea* which is the actual organ of hearing. It has a spiral shape reminiscent of a snail shell and is pointed in the anterior direction. The posterior part of the bony labyrinth has the *vestibule and the semi-circular canals*, which are responsible for equilibrium. The *bony labyrinth* has the

162   *S. R. Savithri*

membranous labyrinth, which is a series of cavities forming a closed system filled with endolymph, a potassium-rich liquid. The *perilymph*, a sodium rich liquid separates the membranous labyrinth from the bony labyrinth. The neurosensory structures involved in hearing and equilibrium are situated in the membranous labyrinth. The *organ of Corti* is situated in the cochlear canal, and the maculae of the utricle and the saccule and the ampullae of the semi-circular canals are located in the posterior section.

The *cochlear canal* is a spiral triangular tube, comprising two and one-half turns, and separates the Scala vestibuli from the Scala tympani. One end of the canal terminates in the spiral ligament, a process of the cochlea's central column, and the other is connected to the bony wall of the cochlea. The *Scala vestibuli* terminates in the oval window and the *Scala tympani* terminates in the round window. These two chambers communicate through the helicotrema, the tip of the cochlea. The inferior surface of the cochlear canal is called the *basilar membrane*. The organ of Corti has *inner* (around 3500) and *outer hair cells* (around 11,500) and is responsible for the transduction of acoustic stimuli. All the auditory information is transduced by these 15,000 hair cells. Of the hair cells, the inner hair cells are of vital importance, because they form synapses with approximately 90% of the 30,000 primary auditory neurons. The inner and outer hair cells are separated from each other by an abundant layer of support cells. The cilia of the hair cells are embedded in the *tectorial membrane*, whose free end is located above the cells. The superior surface of the cochlear canal is formed by *Reisner's membrane*. The bodies of the cochlear sensory cells in the basilar membrane are surrounded by nerve terminals, and their axons (approximately 30,000 in number) form the cochlear nerve. The *cochlear nerve* crosses the inner ear canal and transcends to the central structures of the brain stem. The auditory fibers enter the *temporal lobe*, the part of the cerebral cortex that is responsible for the perception of acoustic stimuli. Figure 84 shows the cross-section of one loop of the cochlea.

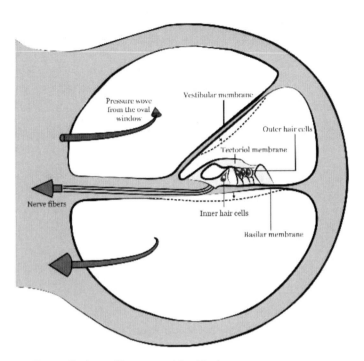

Source: http://www.ilocis.org/documents/chpt11e.htm.

Figure 84. Cross-section of a loop of the cochlea.

The basic function of the ear is hearing. Sound waves passing through the external auditory canal hit the tympanic membrane, which in turn vibrates. This vibration is transmitted to the Malleus, Incus and Stapes. The surface area of the tympanic membrane is around 55 mm^2 and that of the foot of the stapes is around 3.5 mm^2. Hence the surface area of the tympanic membrane is approximately 16 times that of the foot plate of Stapes (55 mm^2/3.5 mm^2). Further there is a lever mechanism of the ossicles. Both these (ratio of the surface area and the lever mechanism of the ossicles) together result in a 22-fold amplification of the sound pressure. Also, the middle ear has a resonance frequency between 1000 to 2000 Hz. Due to this, the transmission ratio is optimal between 1,000 and 2,000 Hz. When the foot of the stapes moves, it causes waves to form in the liquid within the vestibular canal. Because the liquid is incompressible, each inward movement of the foot of the stapes causes an equivalent outward movement of the round window, towards the middle ear. When the ear is exposed to high sound levels, the stapes muscle contracts, protecting the inner ear from high sound levels. This is termed *attenuation reflex*. In addition, the muscles of the middle ear extend the dynamic range of the ear, improve sound localization, reduce resonance in the middle ear, and control air pressure in the middle ear and liquid pressure in the inner ear. Between the frequencies of 250 and 4,000 Hz, the threshold of the attenuation reflex is approximately 80 dB above the hearing threshold and increases by approximately 0.6 dB/dB as the intensity increases. Its latency is 150 ms at threshold and is 24-35 ms in the presence of intense stimuli. At frequencies below the natural resonance of the middle ear, contraction of the middle ear muscles attenuates sound transmission by approximately 10 dB. Because of its latency, the attenuation reflex provides ample protection from noise generated at rates above two to three per second, but not from discrete impulse noise. The speed of sound waves propagating through the ear depends on the elasticity of the basilar membrane. The elasticity of the basilar membrane increases from the base of the cochlea to the tip, and hence the wave velocity decreases. The vibration energy transfer to Reisner's membrane and the basilar membrane is dependent on the frequency. At high frequencies, the wave amplitude is maximum at the base and at low frequencies; it is greatest at the tip. Hence, the point of maximum mechanical excitation in the cochlea is frequency-dependent. The detection of frequency differences is thus based on this phenomenon. Movement of the basilar membrane brings a shear force in the stereo cilia of the hair cells. It also triggers a series of mechanical, electrical and biochemical events responsible for mechanical-sensory transduction and initial acoustic signal processing. The shear forces on the stereo cilia results in opening of the ionic channels in the cell membranes. This in turn modifies the permeability of the membranes and allows the entry of potassium ions into the cells. This entry of potassium ions results in depolarization and the generation of an *action potential*. Neurotransmitters are liberated at the synaptic junction of the inner hair cells which in turn trigger neuronal impulses. These neuronal impulses travel down the afferent fibers of the auditory nerve toward higher centers. The intensity of auditory stimulation depends on the number of action potentials per unit time and the number of cells stimulated. The perceived frequency of the sound depends on the specific nerve fiber groups activated. There is a specific spatial mapping between the frequency of the sound stimulus and the section of the cerebral cortex stimulated.

The inner hair cells, the mechanoreceptors, transform the acoustic signals into electric messages and send it to the central nervous system. However, they are not responsible for the ear's threshold sensitivity and its extraordinary frequency selectivity. The outer hair cells send no auditory signals to the brain. None the less, their function is to selectively amplify mechano-acoustic vibration at near-threshold levels by a factor of approximately 100 (i.e., 40 dB), and therefore facilitate stimulation of inner hair cells. This amplification is thought to be a function of the micromechanical coupling involving the tectorial membrane. The outer hair cells can produce more energy than they receive from external stimuli. They can contract actively at very high frequencies, and thus can function as cochlear amplifiers.

Interference between outer and inner hair cells creates a feedback loop. This permits control of auditory reception, particularly of *threshold sensitivity and frequency selectivity*. Efferent cochlear fibers thus help in reducing cochlear damage caused by exposure to intense acoustic stimuli. Outer hair cells also undergo reflex contraction in the presence of intense high frequency stimuli. The attenuation reflex of the middle ear, active primarily at low frequencies, and the reflex contraction in the inner ear, active at high frequencies, are therefore complementary.

What we learnt in the previous chapters is sound waves through *air conduction*. Sound waves can also be transmitted through the skull which is called *bone conduction*. Two mechanisms for bone conduction are possible. First, compression waves impacting the skull may cause the incompressible perilymph to deform the round or oval window. As already learnt these two windows have differing elasticity, and therefore movement of the endolymph results in movement of the basilar membrane. Second, movement of the ossicles induces movement in the Scala vestibuli only. In this case, movement of the basilar membrane will be a result of the translational movement produced by the inertia. Bone conduction is usually 30-50 dB lower than air conduction.

The *organs of Equilibrium* are responsible for equilibrium of the body. The sensory cells are located in the ampullae of the *semi-circular canals* and the maculae of the *utricle* and *saccule*. These are stimulated by pressure transmitted through the endolymph which results from the movement of the head or body. The cells connect with bipolar cells whose peripheral processes form two tracts, one from the anterior & external *semi-circular canals*, and the other from the posterior semi-circular canal. These two tracts pass the inner ear canal and unite to form the *vestibular nerve*. The nerve passes to the vestibular nuclei in the brainstem and fibers from the vestibular nuclei, in turn, go to the cerebellar centers controlling eye movements, and to the spinal cord. The amalgamation of the vestibular and cochlear nerves forms the 8th *cranial nerve*, also known as the vestibulocochlear nerve.

1.2. Hearing Range for Intensity and Frequency

The human *hearing range* is between 16 to 25,000 Hz. The ability to hear high frequencies declines with age. By the age of 55 the ability to hear in high frequencies reduces. As already learnt, mechanical vibration induces potential changes in the cells of the inner ear, conduction pathways and higher centers. The human ear can perceive frequencies between 16 Hz-25,000 Hz, sound pressures between 20 μPa to 20 Pa (1 Pascal (Pa) = 1 N/m^2 = 10 mbar). The range of sound pressures - 1-million-fold range - which can be perceived is remarkable. The detection thresholds of sound pressure are frequency-dependent. It is lowest at 1,000-6,000 Hz and increases at both lower and higher frequencies. For practical purposes, as we know, the sound pressure level is expressed in decibels (dB), a logarithmic measurement scale corresponding to perceived sound intensity relative to the auditory threshold. Therefore, 20 μPa is equivalent to 0 dB.

The frequency-discrimination threshold or the minimal detectable difference in frequency is 1.5 Hz up to 500 Hz, and 0.3% of the stimulus frequency at higher frequencies. At sound pressures close to the auditory threshold, the sound-pressure-discrimination threshold is approximately 20%. However, differences of as little as 2% may be detected at high sound pressures. If two sounds differ in frequency by a small amount, only one tone will be heard. The perceived frequency of the tone will be halfway between the two tones; but its sound pressure level is variable. A masking effect occurs if two acoustic stimuli have similar frequencies but differ in intensities. Masking will be complete when the difference in sound pressure is large enough and only the loudest sound is perceived.

Localization of acoustic stimuli depends on the detection of the time lag between the arrival of the stimulus at each ear, and, therefore, requires intact bilateral hearing. The smallest detectable time lag is 3×10^{-5} seconds. Screening effect of the head facilitates localization and results in differences in stimulus intensity at each ear.

2. UP-DOWN AND STAIRCASE PROCEDURE OF ESTIMATING MINIMUM AUDIBLE LEVELS

2.1. The Minimum Audible Level

The *minimum audible level* also called as *absolute threshold of hearing* or *auditory threshold* is the minimum sound level of a pure tone that an average human ear with normal hearing can hear when no other sound is present. It is the sound that can just be heard by the organism. It is not a discrete point and is therefore called as the point at which a sound elicits a response a specified percentage of the time.

The *threshold of hearing* is generally reported as the RMS sound pressure of 20 micro Pascals, corresponding to a sound intensity of 0.98 pW/m^2 at 1 atmosphere and 25°C. RMS sound pressure p can be converted to plane wave sound intensity using $I = p^2/pv$, where ρ is the density of air and v is the speed of sound. It is the quietest sound a young human with intact hearing can detect at 1,000 Hz (Gelfand, 1990). The threshold of hearing is frequency-dependent and Johnson (2015) has shown that the ear's

168   *S. R. Savithri*

sensitivity is best at frequencies between 2 kHz and 5 kHz. Pete (2014) reported that the threshold between 2 kHz and 5 kHz may reach as low as −9 dB SPL.

Measurement of the absolute hearing threshold provides basic information about the human auditory system. The methods used to measure the absolute hearing threshold are called *psychophysical methods*. The perception of a physical stimulus (sound) and the human ear's psychological response to the sound is measured, using the psychophysical methods (Hirsh, 1952).

Several psychophysical methods are available to measure absolute threshold. Some variations are there in these methods; but certain aspects are identical. All the methods define *the stimulus* and specify the *manner* in which the participant should *respond*. A sound is presented to the listener and the stimulus level is manipulated in a predetermined pattern. Therefore, the absolute threshold is defined statistically, as an average of all obtained hearing thresholds.

Some methods use a series of trials, and in each trial a 'single-interval "yes"/"no" paradigm' is used. That is sound is present or absent in the single interval, and the listener has to indicate whether he thought the stimulus was there (yes) or not (no). A catch trial, that is a trial in which there is no stimulus, is also presented (Gelfand, 1990).

Before going on to the methods of determining absolute thresholds, let us understand *psychometric function*. In a typical psychometric function, the stimulus level is plotted on the X-Axis and the number of positive responses is plotted on the Y-Axis. Figure 85 shows a typical psychometric function.

Two parameters are of interest in Figure 85. First is the location of the curve, usually defined by the stimulus level corresponding to 50% positive response or X_{50}, the second is the spread of the curve, defined by the distance DL between two conveniently chosen points such as X_{75} (stimulus level at 75% response − 0 in the figure) and X_{50} (stimulus level at 50% response − 2 in the figure). Hence, $X_{75} - X_{50} = 2\text{-}0 = 2$, in this example. In some applications, X_{50} is defined as the *threshold* and DL as the *differential threshold*.

Audibility and Hearing 169

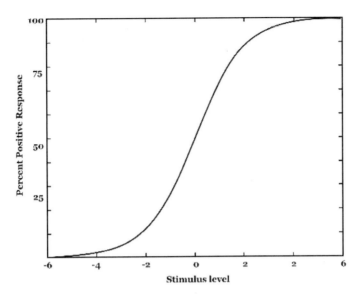

Source: https://en.wikipedia.org/wiki/Psychometric_function.

Figure 85. A typical psychometric function.

Several assumptions are made when using up-down or conventional testing procedures. These assumptions include "(a) the expected proportion of positive responses is a monotonic function of stimulus level, (b) the psychometric function is stationary with time, (c) the psychometric function has a specific parametric form, and (d) responses obtained from the observer are independent of each other and of the preceding stimuli" (Levitt, 1971).

3. CONVENTIONAL OR CLASSICAL METHODS

Classical methods were first described by *Gustav Theodor Fechner* in his work *Elements of Psychophysics* (Hirsh, 1952). Three methods were traditionally used for testing a participant's perception of a stimulus - the *method of limits*, the *method of constant stimuli*, and the *method of adjustment* (Gelfand, 1990).

3.1. Method of Limits

In this method, the tester controls the level of the stimuli. Single-interval *yes/no* paradigm' is used, and there are no catch trials. The trial uses several series of descending and ascending runs. The trial starts with the descending run. Initially a stimulus is presented at a level well above the expected threshold. When the participant responds correctly (yes) to the stimulus, the level of intensity of the sound is decreased by a specific amount and presented again. The same pattern is repeated till the participant stops (no) responding to the stimuli. At this point the descending run is completed and the ascending run starts. In this, the stimulus is first presented well below the threshold and then gradually increased in two decibel (dB) steps until the participant responds. There are no clear margins to 'hearing' and 'not hearing'. Therefore, the threshold for each run is determined as the midpoint between the last audible (yes) and first inaudible level (no). The absolute hearing threshold is calculated as the mean of all obtained thresholds in ascending and descending runs. Figure 86 illustrates a series of descending and ascending runs in the method of limits. In this example, in the first descending trial D1, the participant has responded to 26 dB SPL and stopped responding to 22 dB SPL and therefore D1 = (26 + 22) / 2 = 24 dB SPL. In the same way A1 = 28 dB SPL, D2 = 20 dB SPL and A2 = 28 dB SPL. Therefore, the threshold is equal to (24+28+20+28)/ 4 = 25 dB SPL.

The method of limits helps in estimating the threshold. However, there are some issues related to this method. The anticipation or the participant is aware that there should be a change in the response, or he can choose yes or no only. This anticipation results in better ascending thresholds and worse descending thresholds. Second is the habituation which creates a completely opposite effect. Habituation occurs when the subject becomes accustomed to responding either "yes" in the descending runs and/or "no" in the ascending runs. Because of this, the thresholds are usually raised in ascending runs and improved in descending runs. Third is the step size. Too large a step compromises accuracy of the measurement as the actual threshold is calculated as the average of two stimulus levels. Last, as the tone is always present, "yes" will always be the correct answer (Gelfand, 1990).

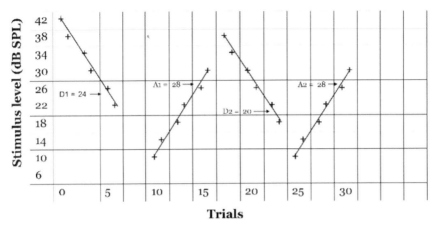

Source: https://www.wikiwand.com/en/Absolute_threshold_of_hearing.

Figure 86. A series of descending and ascending runs in the method of limits.

3.2. Method of Constant Stimuli

In this method, the tester sets the level of stimuli and presents them at completely random order. The participant is expected to respond "yes"/"no" after each presentation. Hence, there are no ascending or descending trials. The stimuli are presented many times at each level. The threshold is defined as the stimulus level at which the subject scored 50% correct. "Catch" trials may be included in this method.

Method of constant stimuli is advantageous than the *method of limits*. As, the stimuli is presented in a random order, the correct answer cannot be predicted by the listener. Further, as there are catch trials, in which there is no tone, "yes" is not always the correct answer. Also, catch trials help to detect the amount of a listener's guessing. The main disadvantage is that a large number of trials are required to measure the threshold, and therefore more time required to complete the test (Gelfand, 1990).

3.3. Method of Adjustment

Method of adjustment has some features of the method of limits in that there are descending, and ascending runs and the listener knows that the stimulus is always present. However, in the method of limits, the tester controls the stimulus but in the method of adjustment, the stimulus is controlled by the listener. The listener reduces the level of the tone until it cannot be detected anymore or increases until it can be heard again. He varies the stimulus level continuously via a dial and the stimulus level is measured by the tester at the end. The threshold is the mean of the just audible and just inaudible levels. Figure 87 illustrates the method of adjustment.

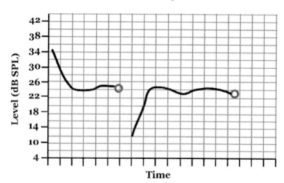

Source: https://www.google.com/search?q=method+of+adjustment&tbm=isch&source =iu&ictx=1&fir=uAwG5E1nlzRluM%253A%252CBRIyJ9xvJo_M1M%252C_& vet=1&usg=AI4_-kS5_KwqCOeXEmRx3FnPbpPxT_c4JQ&sa=X&ved= 2ahUKEwiMkpWZldLiAhUhTY8KHfUADSoQ9QEwAHoECAUQAw#imgrc=- JQSL-2HMb03gM:&vet=1.

Figure 87. Illustration of the method of adjustment.

The method of adjustment has several *biases*. A labelled dial can give cues about the actual stimulus level. To avoid giving cues about the actual stimulus level, the dial must be unlabeled. Apart from anticipation and habituation, stimulus persistence could influence the result from the method of adjustment. In the descending runs, the listener may continue to reduce the level of the sound as if the sound was still audible, while the stimulus is actually well below the actual hearing threshold. In contrast, in the ascending runs, the listener may have persistence of the absence of the stimulus until the hearing threshold is passed by certain amount (Hirsh &Watson, 1996).

3.4. Forced-Choice Methods

In this method, two intervals are presented to a listener, one with a tone and one without a tone. Listener's task is to decide which interval had the tone in it. The number of the intervals can be increased from two. However, it may cause problems as the listener has to remember which interval contained the tone (Gelfand, 1990).

3.5. Adaptive Methods

An adaptive procedure is a procedure in which the stimulus level of a trial is determined by the preceding stimuli and responses. Several psychophysical techniques are adaptive procedures. The von Bekesy technique and the method of limits are two well-known examples. In the classical methods the pattern for changing the stimuli is pre-set; but, in adaptive methods, the listener's response to the previous stimuli decides the level at which a subsequent stimulus has to be presented (Levitt, 1971). Adaptive methods include staircase methods or up-down methods and Bekesy's tracking method.

3.6. Staircase' Methods or Up-Down Methods

The up-down methods of testing are a subset of sequential experiments. A sequential experiment is one in which the course of the experiment is dependent on the experimental data. Two of the sequential experiments have gained attention – (a) those in which the number of observations is determined by the data, and (b) those in which the choice of stimulus levels is determined by the data. The former, first described by Wald in 1947, has some application in psychoacoustics; the latter in general, and the up-down method in particular has found extensive application in psychoacoustics. The simple up-down method is similar to the method of limits in that the stimulus level is decreased after a positive response or increased after a negative response. However, unlike the method of limits, the test is not terminated after the first reversal. It is recommended to continue testing until at least 6 or 8 reversals are obtained (Levitt, 1971). The term *step* refers to the increments by which the stimulus is either increased or decreased. A series of steps in a single direction (ascending or descending) is defined as a run. The stimulus level used in the first trial is referred to as *initial value*.

The *simple '1-down-1-up' method* consists of series of descending and ascending trials runs and turning points or reversals. Reversal means changing from descending to ascending trial. The stimulus level is decreased in the descending trial when the listener responds and increased in the ascending trial when the listener does not respond. After conducting six to eight reversals, the first one is discarded. The threshold is defined as the average of the midpoints of the remaining runs. Levitt (1971) reported that this method provides only 50% accuracy. In order to produce more accurate results, this method can be further *transformed* by increasing the size of steps in the descending runs, for example, '2-down-1-up method', '3-down-1-up methods' (Gelfand, 1990).

3.7. Bekesy's Tracking Method

Bakery's method contains some aspects of classical methods and some of staircase methods. The level of the stimulus is automatically varied at a fixed rate. The listener is instructed to press a button when the stimulus is detectable. Once the listener presses the button, the stimulus level is automatically decreased by the motor-driven attenuator and, on contrary, increased when the button is not pushed. The threshold is thus tracked by the listeners and calculated as the mean of the midpoints of the runs as recorded by the automat (Gelfand, 1990).

4. Minimum Audible Pressure and Field, Missing Six dB and Related Issues

4.1. Minimum Audible Pressure (MAP)

"*Minimum audible pressure* or MAP is the minimum level of a tone which can be presented via headphones to a participant at the minimum threshold of audibility. It is the minimum level which a tone or sound can be produced and then heard by the participant, even when wearing headphones" (Pam, 2013). For a continuous tone of between 2000 and 4000 Hertz, heard by a person with good hearing acuity under laboratory conditions, that is 0.0002 dyne/cm^2 sound pressure and is given the reference level of 0 dB (Pam, 2013).

4.2. Minimum Audible Field (MAF)

"*Minimum audible field* is the threshold before which a tone cannot be heard by a participant. Participants are presented with tones in a sound field without wearing any headphones to better emulate hearing something in a real-life situation. The MAF is the threshold below which a tone or sound cannot be heard" (Pam, 2013).

In terms of amplitude, the eardrum moves about 0.000000001 cm, much less than the wavelength of light. If the ear were any more sensitive, it would have detected the random movements of air molecules. The reference employed is 0 dB; but the threshold of hearing varies considerably with frequencies. It is also called *minimum audible field* (Pam, 2013). In essence MAP and MAF should be the same.

4.3. The Missing Six dB

Sivian and White published an article in 1933 which showed that pressure thresholds at low frequencies using conventional earphones mounted in flat cushions were approximately 6 dB higher than thresholds on the same participants when the sound source was the loud speaker and the participant's ears were not covered. That is, the minimum audible pressure (MAP) differed significantly from the minimum audible field (MAF). No acceptable explanation was provided for this effect. During World War II, loudness balance techniques were used to measure the real ear response of earphones and the attenuation of earphone cushions. The same problem was also observed during these measurements. It was observed that 6 dB more sound pressure was required when equal loudness judgements at low frequencies were made when the source of the sound was conventional earphones compared to when it was a loudspeaker (Beranek, 1949). This problem, whether relating to *thresholds* or *loudness balances*, has been referred to as *the missing 6 dB*. No explanation was available for this. Rudmose (1962) provided some explanation for this phenomenon. The explanation was that physiological noise is generated in the ear canal due to the excitation of the earphone cushion which is tightly coupled to the small volume, approximately 5 cm^3, of the ear canal (Brogden & Miller, 1947). Later research (Rudmose, 1962, 1963) showed that the difference at threshold was due to physiological noise generated in the ear canal by the earphone-cushion-head combination which could be eliminated with a special earphone-coupling system. The suprathreshold differences obtained with loudness balancing were due to a number of procedural and experimental techniques that could be modified to avoid all of the problems of past experimenters. Hence the case of the missing 6 dB was considered closed by the author.

5. AUDITORY THRESHOLD

Auditory threshold refers to the minimum level of sound that can be detected and reported by an organism (Pam, 2013).

5.1. Phon

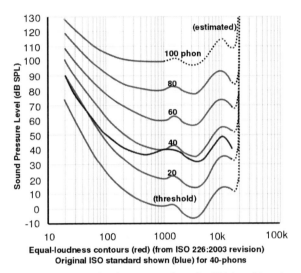

Source: http://www.animations.physics.unsw.edu.au/jw/dB.htm#Loudness.

Figure 88. Equal loudness contours.

While intensity is a physical attribute of a sound what we perceive is loudness (Hartmann, 2004). The *phon* is a unit of loudness level for pure tones. We have learnt about the relationship between sound intensity and sound pressure. Loudness is the subjective perception of sound pressure. The phon was proposed by Stevens in 1936. The number of phon of a sound is the dB SPL of a sound at a frequency of 1 kHz that sounds just as loud. This indicates that 0 phon is the limit of perception, and inaudible sounds have negative phon levels. The *equal-loudness contours* are a way of mapping the dB SPL of a pure tone to the perceived loudness level in phons. The equal-loudness contours on which the phon is based apply only to the perception of pure steady tones; however, tests using octave or third-octave bands of noise show a different set of curves, because of the way in which the critical bands of the human hearing integrate power over varying bandwidths and the human brain sums the various critical bands. An equal-loudness contour is a measure of sound pressure (dB SPL), over the frequency spectrum, for which a listener perceives a constant loudness for pure tones. The unit of measurement for loudness levels is the phon, and is deduced at by reference to equal-loudness contours. Two sine waves of differing frequencies can have equal-loudness level measured in phons, provided they are perceived as equally loud by the average young person without significant hearing impairment. Equal-loudness contours are often referred to as "Fletcher-Munson" curves. The human ear is most sensitive between 2 and 5 kHz, due to the resonance of the ear canal and the transfer function of the ossicles of the middle ear. Fletcher and Munson first measured equal-loudness contours using headphones (1933). Subjects listened to pure tones at various frequencies and over 10 dB increments in stimulus intensity. For each frequency and intensity, the listener also listened to a reference tone at 1 kHz. Fletcher and Munson adjusted the reference tone until the listener perceived that it was the same loudness as the test tone. Loudness, being a psychological quantity, differs between individuals. Hence, Fletcher and Munson averaged their results over all subjects. The lowest equal-loudness contour represents the quietest audible tone or the *absolute threshold of hearing* and the highest contour is the *threshold of pain*. Following this, Churcher and King carried out a second experiment in 1937. But their results were not in consonance with those of Fletcher and Munson. Robinson and Dadson (1956) conducted a more accurate experimental determination which became the basis for a standard (ISO 226) that was considered authoritative until 2003. In response to recommendations in a study coordinated by the Research Institute of Electrical Communication, Tohoku University, Japan, new curves by combining the results of several studies by researchers in Japan, Germany, Denmark, UK, and USA, were derived and standardized as ISO 226:2003. Figure 88 shows equal loudness contours as per ISO 226:2003.

5.2. Sone

The *sone*, proposed by Stevens in 1936, is also a unit of loudness and the sone scale is linear. Doubling the perceived loudness doubles the sone value.

Table 7. Example of loudness in sone, along with sound pressure and SPL

Source of sound	Sound pressure	SPL	Loudness
	Pascal	dB re 20 µPa	Sone
Threshold of pain	100	134	~ 676
Hearing damage during short-term effect	20	120 approx.	~ 256
Jet, 100 m away	6....2000	110...140	~ 128...1024
Hearing damage during long-term effect	$6*10^{-1}$	90 approx.	~ 32
Passenger car, 10 m away	$2\times10^{-2} ... 2\times10^{-1}$	60...80	~ 4...16
TV set at home level, 1 m away	2×10^{-2}	60 approx.	~ 4
normal talking, 1 m away	$2\times10^{-3} ... 2\times10^{-2}$	40...60	~ 1...4
Very calm room	$2\times10^{-4} ... 6\times10^{-4}$	20...30	~ 0.15 ... 0.4
Leaves' noise, calm breathing	6×10^{-5}	10	~ 0.02
Auditory threshold at 1 kHz	2×10^{-5}	0	0

According to Stevens, a loudness of *1 sone* is equivalent to the loudness of a signal at 40 phons, the loudness level of a 1 kHz tone at 40 dB SPL. Phon scale with level in dB, not with loudness, and hence, the sone and phon scales are not proportional. The loudness in sones is, very nearly, a power law function of the signal intensity, with an exponent of 0.3 (Moore, 2007; Herman, 2007). That is each 10 phon increase (or 10 dB at 1 kHz) produces a doubling of the loudness in sones (Hänsler & Schmidt, 2008). At frequencies other than 1 kHz, the loudness level in phons is calibrated according to the frequency response of human hearing, using a set of equal-loudness contours. The loudness level in phons is mapped to loudness in sones using the same power law. Table 7 shows an example of loudness in sone, along with sound pressure and SPL and Table 8 shows a comparison of sone and phon.

S. R. Savithri

Table 8. A comparison of sone and phon

Sone	1	2	4	8	16	32	64	128	25	512	1024
Phon	40	50	60	70	80	90	100	110	120	130	140

Loudness N in sones (for $L_N > 40$ phon) (Fastl & Zwicker, 2007):

$$N = \left(10^{\frac{L_N - 40}{10}} \right)^{0.30103} \approx 2^{\frac{L_N - 40}{10}}$$

or loudness level L_N in phons (for $N > 1$ sone):

$$L_N = 40 + 10 \log_2 (N) \tag{27}$$

Corrections are required at lower levels, near the threshold of hearing.

These formulas are for single-frequency sine waves or narrowband signals. For multi-component or broadband signals, a more elaborate loudness model is essential, which accounts for critical bands. A measurement in sones must be specified in terms of the optional suffix G, which means that the loudness value is calculated from frequency groups, and by one of the two suffixes D (for direct field or free field) or R (for room field or diffuse field).

6. REFERENCE EQUIVALENT THRESHOLD SOUND PRESSURE LEVELS AND HEARING LEVELS

6.1. Reference Equivalent Threshold Sound Pressure Level (RETSPL)

An *audiometer* is a machine used for evaluating hearing acuity. It has a hardware unit connected to a pair of headphones, bone vibrator and a feedback button, and controlled by a standard PC. It is a standard equipment that an audiologist uses. Alternatively, software audiometers are available in several different configurations. A standard computer is used in a screening PC-based audiometer. Usually pure tones at various intensities and frequencies (usually from 250 Hz to 8 k Hz) are given to the subject who has to respond to the pure tone when heard. It is used to determine the hearing ability of the subject. The response of the subject is plotted on a graph which is called *audiogram*.

Audiometric zero refers to the level of a pure tone at a given frequency which is minimally detectable by a person with normal hearing. Audiometric zero is used to calibrate audiometers and therefore, by definition, represents 0 dB HI/HL (hearing level). An audiometric zero represents 0 dB HI or no sound.

RETSPL is the mean value of the equivalent threshold sound pressure levels of large number of ears of normal persons of both sexes aged between 18 and 30 years inclusive, at a specified frequency. The threshold of hearing is expressed for a specified acoustical coupler or artificial ear for a specified type of earphone. The unit is decibel or dB.

Hearing level is the sound pressure level at a specific frequency produced by an audiometer. The reference is audiometric zero and it is measured in decibels.

7. SENSATION LEVELS, THRESHOLD OF PAIN, MOST COMFORTABLE LEVELS

7.1. Sensation Level

Sensation level is the absolute intensity of a sound relative to the absolute threshold of the listener and is measured in decibels. A sensation level of 40 dB indicates that the sound is 40 dB more intense than the faintest sound of the same frequency that the listener can hear.

182 *S. R. Savithri*

7.2. Threshold of Pain

The *threshold of pain* or *pain threshold* is the point at which pain begins to be felt along a curve of increasing perception of a stimulus. It is a subjective phenomenon. A distinction should be maintained between the stimulus and the person's resulting pain perception. An IASP (International Association for the Study of Pain) document defines "pain threshold" as "the minimum intensity of a stimulus that is perceived as painful" (IASP). Traditionally the threshold of pain has been defined, as the least stimulus intensity at which a subject perceives pain. The threshold is the experience of the patient, and the intensity measured is a peripheral event. To reiterate, the stimulus is not pain and cannot be a measure of pain.

The intensity at which a stimulus evokes pain is called, *threshold intensity* (IASP). So, if a hotplate on a person's skin begins to hurt at 42 °C, according to International Association for the Study of Pain, that is the *pain threshold temperature* for that bit of skin at that time. It is not the pain threshold but the temperature at which the pain threshold was crossed. The intensity at which a stimulus begins to evoke pain may vary from individual to individual and for a given individual over time.

Table 9. Threshold of pain and the corresponding sound pressure

Sound pressure level	Sound pressure
120 dB SPL	20 Pa
130 dB SPL	63 Pa
134 dB SPL	100 Pa
137.5 dB SPL	150 Pa
140 dB SPL	200

Pain threshold pressure is the pressure at which sound becomes painful for a listener person at that time. The threshold pressure for sound varies with frequency and is dependent on age. People who have been exposed to more noise/music usually have a higher threshold pressure (Barry, 1999). Prolonged exposure to sound at levels evoking pain can cause physical damage, and leads to hearing impairment. Though the upper limit for a

Audibility and Hearing 183

tolerable intensity varies, naive listeners reach a limit at about 125 dB SPL and experienced listeners at 135 to 140 dB of tolerance. Table 9 shows the threshold of pain and the corresponding sound pressure.

7.3. Most Comfortable Listening Level (MCL)

Most comfortable listening level is the level at which a listener finds listening most comfortable and the unit is dB. Running speech or connected discourse is usually used for measurement of MCL and MCL is a very useful test routinely used for hearing aid trial. The listener has to indicate the level at which listening is found to be most comfortable. Usually multiple trials are used as MCL is not an absolute single value but a range. It is a range because people most often want sounds a little louder or a little softer. Whether it is the most comfortable level or a most comfortable range, it is recorded on the audiogram along with the material used. MCL should not be confused with the level at which a listener achieves maximum intelligibility. MCL is useful, but not for determining the maximum intelligibility.

7.4. Uncomfortable Listening Level (UCL)

The *uncomfortable listening level* is the level at which a listener finds listening most uncomfortable and the unit is dB. The listener has to indicate the level at which listening is found to be most uncomfortable. UCL is found out by using running speech. However, the instructions for this test can definitely influence the outcome, as uncomfortable level for some individuals may not really be their UCL; but it might be a preference for listening at a softer level. Therefore, it is important to make the patient understand as to what you mean by uncomfortably loud. UCL is used to estimate the dynamic range for speech which is defined as the difference between the UCL and the speech reception threshold. In normal hearing individuals, this range is usually 100 dB or more; UCL is reduced in ears with sensorineural hearing loss.

184   *S. R. Savithri*

7.5. Acceptable Noise Level (ANL)

Acceptable Noise Level is the amount of background noise that a listener is willing to accept while listening to speech (Nabelek, Tucker, & Letowski, 1991). ANL is a test of noise tolerance and is shown to be related to the successful use of hearing aids and to potential benefit with hearing aids (Nabelek, Freyaldenhoven, Tampas, Burchfiel, & Muenchen, 2006). It uses the MCL and a measure of background noise level (BNL). A recorded speech passage is presented to the listener in the sound field to arrive at MCL. The noise is then introduced to the listener and increased till the person is able to tolerate or "put up with" the noise but can hear the story in the speech passage. The ANL is calculated as the difference between the MCL and the BNL. Individuals who obtain very low scores on the ANL are considered to be successful hearing aid users or good candidates for hearing aids. Those who have very high scores are considered unsuccessful users or poor hearing aid candidates.

CONCLUSION

This chapter covered hearing mechanism, the basic concepts related to hearing and its measurements as it is important to understand hearing mechanism before learning concepts related to hearing and its measurement. It further covered the range of frequency and intensity that the human ear can perceive. For a better appreciation of the readers the chapter included procedures for estimation of audible levels and various methods within these procedures. Among the concepts of hearing, definitions of Minimum audible pressure and field, Missing six dB and related issuessre introduced. The other scales to measure loudness namely phon and sone, and the Audiometric zero, Reference equivalent threshold sound pressure levels and hearing levels, Sensation levels, Threshold of pain, Most comfortable levels, Uncomfortable Listening Level (UCL), and Acceptable Noise Level (ANL) were discussed. For a detailed description, the reader can refer to other books provided in the references.

REFERENCES

Barry, T. 1999. *Handbook for Acoustic Ecology.* (2nd Ed.). ARC Publications, World Soundscape Project, Simon Fraser University.

Beranek, L. L. 1949. *Acoustic Measurements.* New York: Wiley, 731-755.

Brogden, W. J., and Miller, G. A. 1947. "Physiological Noise Generated under Earphone Cushions." *J. Acoust Soc. Amer.*, 19, 620

Churcher, B. G., and King, A. J. 1937. "The performance of noise meters in terms of the primary standard." *J. Inst. Electr. Eng.* 81, 57–90.

Fastl, H. and Zwicker, E. 2007. *Psychoacoustics: facts and models* (3rd Ed.). Berlin/Heidelberg: Springer. p. 207.

Fletcher, H. and Munson, W. A. 1933. "Loudness, its definition, measurement and calculation." *J. Acoust. Soc. Amer.,* 5, 82-108.

Gelfand, S. A. 1990. *Hearing: An introduction to psychological and physiological acoustics.* (2nd Ed.). New York and Basel: Marcel Dekker Inc.

Gelfand, S. A. 2009. *Essentials of Audiology* (3rd Ed.). New York: Thieme Medical Publishers, Inc.

Gelfand, S. A. 2009. *Hearing: An Introduction to Psychological and Physiological Acoustics.* New York: Taylor & Francis.

Gold, B., and Morgan. N. 2002. *Speech and Audio Signal Processing,* New York: John Wiley & Sons.

Hänsler, H. and Schmidt, G. 2008. *"Speech and audio processing in adverse environments."* Edited by H. Hänsler, and G. Schmidt. Berlin/Heidelberg: Springer. 299.

Hartmann, W. M. 2004. *Signals, Sound, and Sensation,* American Institute of Physics Series in Modern Acoustics and Signal Processing.

Herman, I. P. 2007. *Physics of the Human Body.* New York: Springer. 613.

Hirsh, I. J. 1952. *The Measurement of Hearing.* New York: McGraw-Hill.

Hirsh, I. J., and Watson C. S. 1996. "Auditory Psychophysics and Perception." *Annu. Rev. Psychol.* 47: 461-84.

IASP. *IASP Pain Terminology.* IASP Press. Retrieved from https://www.iasp-pain.org/Education/Content.aspx?ItemNumber=1698 #Pain. Accessed February 12.

186   *S. R. Savithri*

ISO 226:2003. Retrieved from https://www.iso.org/standard/34222.html. Accessed February 12.

Johnson, K. 2015. *Acoustic and Auditory Phonetics* (3rd Ed.). UK: Wiley-Blackwell.

Ken'ichiro Masaoka, Kazuho Ono, and Setsu Komiyama. 2001. "A measurement of equal-loudness level contours for tone burst." *Acoustical Science and Technology*, Vol. 22, No. 1, 35–39.

Levitt, H. 1971. Transformed up-down methods in psychoacoustics. *J. Acoust. Soc. Amer.* 49, 467-477.

Martin, F. N., and Clark, J. G. 2015. *Introduction to Audiology* (12th Ed.). New Jersey: Pearson Education, Inc.

Moore, B. C. J. 2007. *Cochlear hearing loss: physiological, psychological and technical issues* (2nd Ed.). New Jersey: John Wiley & Sons.

Nabelek, A. K., Tucker, F. M., and Letowski, T. R. 1991. "Toleration of background noises: relationship with patterns of hearing aid use by elderly persons." *J Speech Hear Res.*, 34(3):679-85.

Nabelek, A. K., Freyaldenhoven, M. C., Tampas, J. W., Burchfiel, S. B., and Muenchen, R. A. 2006. "Acceptable noise level as a predictor of hearing aid use." *J Am Acad Audiol.* 17(9):626-39.

Nave, C. R. 2006. *Threshold of Pain.* HyperPhysics. SciLinks. Department of Physics and Astronomy, Georgia State University, Atlanta, Georgia. Retrieved from http://hyperphysics.phy-astr.gsu.edu/hbase/Sound/intens.html. Accessed February 12.

Newby, H. A., and Popelka, G. R. 1992. *Audiology* (6th Ed). New Jersey: A Simon & Schuster Company.

Norton Canfield cited in H. A. Newby, and G. R. Popelka. 1992. *Audiology* (6th Ed). New Jersey: A Simon & Schuster Company.

Pam, M.S. 2013. "Minimal Audible Prerssure (MAP)." in *PsychologyDictionary.org*, April 7, 2013, https://psychology dictionary.org/minimal-audible-pressure-map/. Accessed February 12.

Pete, J. R. 2014. "What's the quietest sound a human can hear?" (PDF). University College London.

Audibility and Hearing

Priemer, R. 1991) *Introductory Signal Processing (Advanced Series in Electrical and Computer Engineering) (v. 6)*. Teaneck, New Jersey: World Scientific Pub Co Inc.

Rabiner, L. R., and Schafer, R. W. 1978. *Digital processing of speech signals*, New Jersey: Prentice-Hall Inc.

Robinson, D. W., and Dadson, R. S. 1956. "A re-determination of the equal-loudness relations for pure tones." *Br. J. Appl. Phys.* 7, 166–181.

Rudmose, W. 1962. "Pressure vs free field thresholds at low frequencies." *Proc. 4th Int. Congr. Acoust.*, Copenhagen, Paper H52.

Rudmose, W. 1963. "On the lack of agreement between earphone pressures and loudspeaker pressures for loudness balances at low frequencies." *J. Acoust. Soc. Amer.* 35, 1906.

Rudmose. W. 1982. "The case of the missing 6 dB." *J. Acoust. Soc. Amer.* 71 (3), 650-659.

Sivian, L. J., and White, S. D. 1933. "On minimum audible sound fields." *J. Acoust. Soc. Amer.* 4, 288.

Stevens, S. S. 1936. Cited in William M. Hartmann. 2004. *Signals, Sound, and Sensation*, American Institute of Physics. ISBN 1-56396-283-7.

Chapter 5

INTRODUCTION TO SPEECH-LANGUAGE PATHOLOGY AND AUDIOLOGY

INTRODUCTION

Having learnt about basic concepts of Speech-Language Pathology and Audiology, it is important to appreciate the predecessors who contributed to the growth of these fields. Therefore, this chapter covers historical aspects of the field of speech-language pathology and audiology. It includes development of speech and language pathology and audiology in Indian and global context. In the Indian contexts, Institutions for the field, the Indian Speech and Hearing Association, Journals like Journal of the All India Institute of Speech & Hearing, Journal of the Indian Speech & Hearing Association, and Government regulatory bodies like Rehabilitation Council of India are introduced. In the Global context, American Speech Association, The American Academy of Speech Correction, and the Journal of Speech Disorders are covered. The chapter has introduced the important professionals who contributed to the growth of the fields. Under the development of Audiology, Military origin, Community origin, and University origin and services of an audiologist are covered. The development of the fields in other countries is also covered. The

190   *S. R. Savithri*

interdisciplinary nature of speech-language pathology and audiology are introduced owing to the wide range of services by the professionals.

In the next part of the chapter, development of instrumentation in Speech Pathology both Indian and western origin is introduced. In the Indian origin *Pa:n.ini* (4th century BCE) and his classification of speech sounds and *Bhartṛhari* (5th century CE) on the earliest theory of speech perception are covered in detail. The instrumentations included Helmholtz resonator to ERPs by professionals from varying fields such as a Psychophysicist, a Phonetician and Linguist, a Speech Pathologist, a Physiologic Psychologist, an Electrical Engineer, and an ENT specialist. Development of instrumentation in Audiology includes tuning fork, acuity meter to OAE and ERP by various professionals such as Psychologist, Physicist, and biophysicist. Further development of hearing aids - Akouphone to digital hearing aids, and cochlear implants are included.

The last part of the chapter covers scope of Practice in Speech-Language Pathology and Audiology taken from the Indian Speech & Hearing Association website (http://www.ishaindia.org.in/pdf/Scope_of_ Practice.pdf).

1. HISTORICAL ASPECTS OF THE FIELD OF SPEECH-LANGUAGE PATHOLOGY

Knowledge of history can provide lessons from the past, predictions for the future, and a perspective for a better understanding of current theories and practices. It also helps to build introspection for clinical practice, and makes one understand that several theories and methods remain unaltered, while some may be reframed or replaced with new theories and methods. A historical and outside perspective can offer clinicians a way to evaluate their practices, new dimensions from which to view their taken-for-granted ideas and practices, and strength to critically evaluate and change the practices (O'Neill, 1980).

Introduction to Speech-Language Pathology and Audiology 191

One could observe statements about speech and language disorders starting from 3000 A. D. in ancient literature belonging to India, Mesopotamia, Greece, Rome, Egypt and other countries. In fact, information on the origin and development of speech and language, speech production, normality of speech and language, and disorders of speech and language and their treatment are available in ancient Sanskrit literature. However, most of the speech and language disorders were treated medically and a separate field of speech-language pathology did not exist.

In 1770 Gesner described the symptoms of a patient, KD, who had what today we call as jargon aphasia. The patient's problem, according to Gesner, was his inability to associate images with their verbal symbols. He called it verbal amnesia. Crichton, in 1778, published a two-volume text on mental derangements, which included disorders of aphasia, ranging from simple word-finding difficulties to a description of Wernicke's aphasia.

Speech-language pathology had its first origin in elocution (speech perfection) arising from the 18th century in England. Toward the end of the eighteenth century, there was a movement in Europe to create more humane treatments for people with disabilities. Two famous people with stuttering, Moses Mendelssohn and Erasmus Darwin, wrote about their speech problem in positive ways. Darwin considered his stuttering as a gift that trained him to speak concisely and directly to the point. He viewed stuttering as an approach avoidance conflict involving fear and the need to talk. In his theory, this conflict arose from a break in the associations between volition and the muscular movement of articulation. Darwin recommended therapy that involved practicing stuttered words and developing a "carelessness about the opinions of others" (Rieber & Wollock, 1977). Eighteenth century public schools in United States of America included instruction in literacy, grammar, and public speaking or elocution. In the 18th century, institutions of higher education started in America with Yale University, established in 1701, Princeton University in 1746 and the University of Pennsylvania in 1791.The curricula of these universities emphasized rhetoric. For example, the curriculum devised by Benjamin Franklin for the University of Pennsylvania included grammar, reading, public speaking, and writing. The

18th century America witnessed the beginning of special segregated institutions for people with disabilities.

Jean Marc Gaspard Itard (1775-1838), a French physician and educator, worked with a 10-year boy, Victor, who was found in the wild, who later was called *The wild boy of Aveyron.* Itard believed that any child could be taught anything. One of his goals for Victor was to teach speech by using imitation. Sense training was considered important for teaching and Itard's methods included stimulating vision, hearing, taste, and smell and working on eye-hand coordination. Victor improved and could read and speak a few words, interpret and execute simple commands, and display emotional attachment to his caregivers. Itard stopped working with Victor and started developing educational programs for those who are deaf and hearing impaired. Itard's writings about Victor was an influential treatise for later teachers working with children who were diagnosed as mentally retarded (Scheerenberger, 1983). Itard's student Edward Seguin systemized Itard's methods and called them Physiological method (Seguin, 1866). In 1850, Seguin moved to the United States and became a leader in the education of those with mental retardation.

Most speech therapies of the 18th century were driven by the medical model. None the less, not everyone based their therapy and education on a medical model. The British elocutionist John Thelwall disputed that most speech and language problems could be remediated without resorting to medical therapies. Thelwal therapies included exercises to stretch the tissue associated with "tongue tie," phonetic placement, prosody and public speaking. Thus the 18th century Europe and America explored categorization of different types of diseases and disabilities including diseases underlying to speech disorders. Among the notable figures who had considerable impact on the next century's developments affecting the communicatively impaired in America were Benjamin Franklin, John Thelwall, and Jean Marc Itard.

Some elocutionists practicing in the early 19th century saw communication disorders as within their scope of interest and practice. Late in the 19th century, they began to organize themselves into a professional group and a journal, *The Voice*, devoted to topics on elocution and speech

Introduction to Speech-Language Pathology and Audiology 193

correction was established in 1879 by Edgar S. Werner, the National Association of Elocutionists was founded in 1892. A handful of university programs were started to train people to become elocutionists. It was this budding professional group that was to initiate the field of speech correction later.

Between 1870 until the start of the first world war in 1914, several individuals thought that there were some common things among them and found the need to (1) determine qualifications for professionals; (2) identify a profession's jurisdiction; (3) establish ways for obtaining monopoly over the activities that fell within the jurisdiction; and (4) carry out a scientific program to build a knowledge base for assessing professional expertise. Professions that reorganized or formed themselves in this period included medicine, special education, and speech correction. Each dealt with the four concerns in its own way.

2. HISTORICAL ASPECTS IN THE FIELD OF AUDIOLOGY

Audiology is the *study of hearing and its disorders*. Several fields have contributed to the growth of the field. The field of Audiology rose from two fields – *Speech Pathology and Otology* (Newby & Popelka, 1992). As already described Speech Pathology is a field dealing with the identification, diagnosis and rehabilitation of persons with speech and language disorders. Otology is a medical field and a division of Otorhinolaryngology which refers to the study of diseases of ear, nose, and throat. The armed forces, for the benefit of hearing-impaired persons, combined two fields of Speech Pathology and Otology during the Second World War Rehabilitation of these persons, which required the team work of medical and nonmedical specialists. Some of the nonmedical specialists recruited were teachers of the deaf with training and experience in the field of Speech Pathology and Speech Correction. They started developing tests of hearing function, selection of hearing aids and development of rehabilitative techniques. Thus, with the cooperation of the two fields of Speech Pathology and Otology, the new field of audiology was created. The word Audiology did not exist until

194   *S. R. Savithri*

World War II. Raymond Carhart, a Speech Pathologist who was recruited for aural rehabilitation by the army, and Norton Canfield, an Otologist, who was the consultant to the war department coined the term Audiologist (Newby & Popelka, 1992). There are some disputes about the time when the term was coined. However, the term has become popular from the date it was coined by Carhart and Canfield.

Though the parents of Audiology are Speech Pathology and Otology, there exist other relatives of the family. The medical relatives include pediatrics, gerontology, psychiatry, neurology and neurosurgery and more recently electronics and information technology. The non-medical relatives are psychology, physics and education.

3. DEVELOPMENT OF SPEECH AND LANGUAGE PATHOLOGY AND AUDIOLOGY: INDIAN AND GLOBAL CONTEXT

3.1. Indian Context

Deaf schools were in existence in India to provide speech therapy and sign language to deaf children. Dr. Martin F Palmer, Director, Institute of Logopedics, under Department of Health, Education & Welfare, University of Kansas, Wichita, was invited by the Government of India in 1963. Following his visit, the Institute of Logopedics was started in the year 1965 in Mysore by the Ministry of Health & Family Planning, Govt. of India as a subordinate office under DGHS. Natesh Ratna was appointed as Officer on Special duty by the DGHS, Ministry of Health and Family Planning, Govt. of India. A 2-year master's programme in speech and hearing was initiated in the year 1966 quickly followed by a 3-year bachelors programme in speech and hearing. At around the same time a 2-year Audiology & Speech Language Therapy program was started, at Topiwala National Medical College and BYL Nair Charitable Hospital in Mumbai and Ramesh K Oza took the responsibility to conduct the programme. The Institute of

Introduction to Speech-Language Pathology and Audiology 195

Logopedics at Mysore was registered as a society on 10.10.1966 under the name All India Institute of Speech & Hearing and became the nodal agency for all speech and hearing work in India since then. In the 1980s, other government institutions and centers like All India Institute of Medical Sciences, New Delhi, and Ali Yavar Jung National Institute for the Hearing Impaired, Mumbai started offering graduate courses in speech and hearing, and clinical services. Following these, the Regional Rehabilitation Centers with their branches in Chennai (Tamil Nadu), Hyderabad (Andhra Pradesh), Cuttack (Orissa), and New Delhi started catering to the clinical needs clientele speaking various languages of India. In early 1990's, Non-Government Organizations started institutions (for example Institute of Speech & Hearing at Bangalore, and M V Shetty Institute of Speech & Hearing at Mangalore) to offer undergraduate courses initially and Postgraduate courses later. In the mid of 1990's other Government organizations started Institutions like National Institute of Speech & Hearing at Trivandrum and ICCONS at Trivandrum. As on date there are about 56 Institutions (retrieved from http://rehabcouncil.nic.in) offering academic programmes in the field of speech and hearing in India. These Institutions have generated around 1700 manpower in the field that are catering to the needs of persons with communication disorders.

Forming an association of speech and hearing was first discussed on the 4th of April 1966, at the First All India Workshop on Speech and Hearing Problems at Vellore. A decision of forming an association of Speech and Hearing was taken at Pune in 1967 at the Annual conference of the *Association of Otolaryngologists of India*. The *Indian Speech & Hearing Association (ISHA) came into existence on 15th December 1967*. It was registered under the Mysore Societies Registration Act, 1960 on 15.12.1967. The association has its central office at All India Institute of speech and Hearing, Manasagangothri, Mysore-57006. The first conference was a part of the Annual conference of the Association of Otolaryngologists of India and was held in Calcutta in 1968. ISHA was under the Association of Otolaryngologists of India till 1977 and in 1978 it became independent and held its first independent conference in Mysore. ISHA also has a Journal of

196   *S. R. Savithri*

its own named *Journal of the Indian speech and Hearing Association.* (retrieved from http://www.ishaindia.org.in/aboutus.html).

The *Rehabilitation Council of India* (RCI) was set up as a registered society in 1986.On September,1992 the RCI Act was enacted by Parliament and it became a Statutory Body on 22 June 1993.The Act was amended by Parliament in 2000 to make it more broad based. The mandate of RCI is to regulate and monitor services given to persons with disability, to standardize syllabi and to maintain a Central Rehabilitation Register of all qualified professionals and personnel working in the field of Rehabilitation and Special Education. (Retrieved from http://rehabcouncil.nic.in).

3.2. Global Context

3.2.1. Speech-Language Pathology

Like for their sister professions, practitioners and researchers in the field of "speech correction," realized a need for an organization for them. These specialists were from various disciplines. For example, Smiley Blanton in medicine and psychiatry; Walter Babcock Swift with medicine and education; Edwin Twitmyer a clinical psychologist, with a specialty in speech disorders; Edgar S. Werner with elocutionists. Some of these professionals started to meet together at the conventions of one parent profession, *American Speech Association.* They worked to establish professional qualifications, practice jurisdiction, practice monopoly, and scientific grounding for those entering and working in the field of speech correction. The *American Academy of Speech Correction*, approved in 1926, aimed "to raise existing standards of practice among workers in the field of speech correction" (Anon, 1927). The University of Iowa started the Department of Speech. In 1936, the group began its own journal, the *Journal of Speech Disorders.*

During 1925, the National Association of Teachers of Speech (NATS) met in New York City, and started with the *American Academy of Speech Correction* to promote scientific, organized work in the field of speech correction. The name of the society changed to American Society

Introduction to Speech-Language Pathology and Audiology   197

for the Study of Disorders of Speech (1927), American Speech Correction Association (1934), American Speech and Hearing Association (1947), and American Speech-Language-Hearing Association (1978) (https://www.asha.org/about/history/).

In the 19th century, in America, three trends led to the need for the first speech-language pathology professionals which worked together to form a common pathway that eventually guided the formation of the profession in 1925. The first trend was the *elocution movement* which was set up to work with orators, politicians, singers, preachers, actors, and non-specialists who wanted to improve their speaking, orating, or singing. The noteworthy names include Andrew Comstock and Alexander Graham Bell. Alexander Graham Bell opened a School of Vocal Physiology in Philadelphia, in 1872. The influence of Charles Darwin, the work of Paul Broca, and Carle Wernicke on brain and language lead to establishment of the first academic psychology programs in the Europe and the United States. All these influences created a scientific revolution, and lead to the founding of American Speech and Hearing Association in 1925. Edward Lee Travis called a meeting at his house in Iowa City, Iowa to form this new organization. Some of these professionals had expertise from having cured their own speech problems. James Sonnett Greene described agitophasia (cluttering) and agitographia (illegible writing involving missing letters and syllables). He associated these to brain centers. Brain localizations started. For example, oral language disabilities (word deafness) were thought of as problems within the auditory word center and reading problems as breakdowns in the visual word center (word blindness). These were coined & identified by Samuel Torrey Orton (1925), a Psychiatrist at the University of Iowa, and Mildred MaGinnis (1929), a teacher at Central Institute for the Deaf, St. Louis. Samuel Torrey Orton also researched on hemispheric localization. Edward Wheeler Scripture established a laboratory at Yale University and collected all techniques to measure different aspects of speech production and acoustic perception. He used Kymograph to record airflow and articulation during the speech production, plaster molds of the alveolar ridge to get tongue impressions during alveolar consonant production, tongue – palate impressions to obtain impressions during the production of palatal consonants. Floyd Summer Muckey (1858 – 1930), a nose and throat specialist was the first to analyze tone and to make a photo of the vocal cords in action. George Oscar Russell (1890 – 1962) at the Universities of Iowa and Chicago invented palatograph where dynamic movements of the tongue were revealed through bends in aluminium foil and used X-Ray for examining the articulatory positions during vowel production. Further, Carl Emil Seashore (1866-1949) invented and patented Iowa Pitch Range audiometer, Tonoscope, Chronoscope, Time-sense apparatus, and Stimulus Key.

Thus, in the USA, during the 20th century, during the first 45 years, the profession established itself as a separate independent from medicine. However, therapy included both medical and educational approaches. Therapies focused on speech sounds to word sequences, sensory and motor training. Clinicians used drilling of the sounds in sensory training and used physical placement of articulators & tongue exercises in motor training. During the next 20 years, therapies became more wholistic and aimed at less observable aspects of speech and language. The focus of therapy was beginning with words, symbol formation and inner language. Further, visual and auditory modalities were used in therapies. During the next 10 years, the clinicians developed programs for teaching phonological and grammatical rules. Therapies were behaviorally oriented and used repetitive practice on discrete items. Recently, the clinical practice concerns as how messages are used, & how they fit into the situational and cultural contexts of everyday life communication. The clinical services were also delivered in classrooms, homes and community settings (retrieved from http://www.acsu.buffalo. edu/~duchan/history_summary.html).

The important professionals included Alexander Graham Bell, Melville Bell, Paul Broca, Dorothea McCarthy, Samuel Orton, Carl Emil Seashore, Lee Edward Travis, Charles Van Riper, Carl Wernicke, Robert West, among others.

Introduction to Speech-Language Pathology and Audiology   199

3.2.2. Audiology

3.2.2.1. Military Origin of the Development of Audiology

The field of Audiology developed directly from the Military. Initially 3 aural rehabilitation centers were established by the army at Borden General Hospital, Chikasha, Oklahoma; Hoff General Hospital, Santa Barbara, California, and Deshon General Hospital, Butler, Pennsylvania. These were of tremendous help in aural rehabilitation and proved themselves. The military requested help from college and university speech clinics, teachers of lip reading & deaf, and psychologists to develop a program of rehabilitation. As the aural rehabilitation programs were the responsibility of medical professionals, initially they were under the physicians – ENT specialists. The first and major responsibility of the aural rehabilitation center was to identify whether causality would benefit from medical or surgical care. Some speech specialist started developing and administering tests to evaluate the function of hearing. They were termed *acoustic physicians* who later were called *audiologists*. Patients who could not be medically treated were placed in the rehabilitation program which was basically to select the hearing aid, impart speech reading, auditory training and counselling. As on date the Federal government of USA continues to provide audiological services to active Military personnel (Newby & Popelka, 1992).

Immediately after World War II, several of them wanted continued aural rehabilitation services. The Veterans Administration established audiology clinics in several regional offices and veterans' hospitals and distributed hearing aids as compensation (Newby & Popelka, 1992).

3.2.2.2. Community Origin

The *Military aural rehabilitation centers* were so effective to be impressed by the administration, which in turn was the cause for starting such clinic for civilians. Though Otologists were responsible for aural rehabilitation, as they did not have the desire or the time, the clinical program was shifted to *acoustic physicians* or *audiologists*. The major responsibility of the Veteran centers was to do audiometric testing and hearing aid selection. The *civilian canters* also focused on the same. However, neither were the civilians willing to devote several weeks for training nor could they be commanded to do so. Therefore, several modifications in the aural rehabilitation program had to be done. The civilian centers slowly evolved in to *community hearing centers* to provide professional services to the needy referred from medical professionals. Some of these community hearing centers were affiliated to the *National Association of Hearing and Speech Action* known formerly as *American Hearing Society*. However, some centers were non-profit, private sponsored agencies. These community hearing centers, to continue their existence, had to prove themselves with high quality professional services (Newby & Popelka, 1992).

3.2.2.3. University Origin

Initially, before the Second World War, *speech clinics* in existence treated speech defects such as stuttering, aphasia, voice problems, articulation problems, cleft palate, and speech training for the hard of hearing. The necessity of handling hearing handicapped veterans following the Second World War gave a thrust to colleges and universities to develop programs and allied medical services in the field of Audiology. In 1947, the *American Speech Correction Association* changed its name to *American Speech and Hearing Association* and its official publication *Journal of Speech Disorders* was changed to *Journal of Speech and Hearing Disorders*. In parallel the name *speech clinic* was changed to *speech and hearing clinic*. By 1950, *training program in Audiology* started in most of the colleges and universities which were previously offering training programming in the field of speech correction. Thus, 5 years after the termination of World War II, the importance of audiology as a separate discipline from speech pathology was recognized (Newby & Popelka, 1992).

Also, a development occurred in the medical settings. To start with, audiological services in medical services were located in hospitals and audiology served such patients who were referred by physicians only. In a hospital setting the audiology program was with department of otolaryngology, or neurology, or pediatrics, or physical medicine. However,

Introduction to Speech-Language Pathology and Audiology 201

a variety of medical settings, such as inpatient, outpatient, single physician's office, group medical practices and so on, had emerged. This enabled the audiological program in other settings also. Other settings including industrial, school, commercial settings, and private practice also evolved (Newby & Popelka, 1992).

3.2.2.4. Services

An audiologist has two services – diagnostic and rehabilitation. Diagnostic audiology includes assessing the degree of hearing of a patient, differential diagnosis, and analyzing the hearing problems. Pure tone audiometry, speech audiometry, immittance, evoked responses and reflex measurements aid an audiologist to measure the hearing ability. Assessment of hearing problems in infants and children, who are most often non-cooperative patients, has necessitated the development of tests specific to this population. Rehabilitation audiology covers all services that are not diagnostic and includes selection, fitting and dispensing of hearing aids, speech reading, auditory training, and hearing aid orientation.

Two educational programs started around the year 1956 in Canada. By 1961, there were about 100 and 120 speech therapists and audiologists practicing in Canada. The Manitoba Speech and Hearing Association was started in the year 1958 and women were members of the association who assessed other members and voted unanimously to initiate legislation to regulate practice in the field. Led by Isabel Richard the first legislation to regulate the professions in all of North America was enacted in 1961. The legislation required all practicing in the province to be registered by the association and the bill is still in force.

In India, as already mentioned speech & hearing programmes and services started in the year 1966. Audiology, as a profession is recognized by the Rehabilitation Council of India, and the University of Mysore from the year 2003.

3.2.2.5. Other Countries

3.2.2.5.1. Europe

The temples of Mesopotamia, and Greek supported blind and deaf apart from others with disabilities by providing jobs. It is hard to find mention of persons with communication disorders in the literature of Mesopotamia. However, Hittite king, Mursilis (1344 – 1320) described his loss of speech which was found on the inscriptions of a clay tablet. Rehabilitation included oral training, prayers and sacrifices to god, physical exercises, baths & fresh air, and speech exercises involving the tongue & voice by Greeks.

Aesop (6th Century B C) was considered to have a speech problem. Aristotle (384 – 322 B C) wrote about speech disorders; Caelius Aurelianus (5th Century A D) from Rome separated speech problems from voice problems. Claudius (10 B C – 54 A D), the Roman emperor was known to have cerebral palsy. Demosthenes (384 – 322 B C), a Greek orator is believed to have overcome his speech problem. Soranus of Ephesus (98 B C – 138 A D) differentiated between speech disorders caused by tongue paralysis and other causes.

Albertus Magnus (1193 – 1282), a German philosopher wrote about voice and articulation. Balbulus (840 – 912), a Swiss musician teacher had a speech problem. Eustacia (6th Century A D), a mystic, helped cure a woman with paralysis of the tongue. Peter of Abano (1250 – 1316), an Italian Philosopher, astronomer, and medical authority, wrote on various aspects of speech & hearing problems. Rudolph Agricola (1444 - 1485), a Dutch scholar, taught deaf person to communicate orally and in writing.

In the *early modern period,* a dramatic change happened in all fields. Insights on anatomy, blood circulation helped to create new ideas about origins and treatment of communication disorders resulting from stroke. Hieronymous Mercurialis (1530 – 1606) studied speech disorders which led to medical look at such disorders, provided diagnostic criteria, possible etiologies, and remediation. A move to use Latin as the language of literacy and oratory, led to universal language movement which helped in accessing languages. This move also created interest in teaching speech to the deaf. Alternate and augmented means of communication, including sign language,

Introduction to Speech-Language Pathology and Audiology 203

lip reading, written language and pictures, were designed and taught to non-verbal children.

The 18th century saw some advances in the field such as categorization of diseases & disabilities, and diseases underlying speech disorders. The French and American revolutions led to a need for the creation of equal opportunities for the poor, the women, and for the non-enfranchised including persons with speech problems. Efforts were made to standardize language and to promote it as a way for everyone to communicate. One of the major things that happened in the 18th century were studies on structure of speech and language, aspects of the language system – phonetics, prosody, lexicon, morphology, grammar -. Speech and educational therapies, such as sensation – based learning theories, were developed by Jean Itard.

3.2.2.5.2. Saudi Arabia

The first audiology and SLP program was established at King Saud University in 1987. The Saudi Society of Speech-Language Pathology and Audiology (SSSPA) was officially established in 2003. Currently, three Saudi universities offer three undergraduate programs and only one graduate program in audiology and/or speech-language pathology. Of these two are government and one is private. King Saud University offers a duel degree undergraduate program in speech and hearing rehabilitation, Princess Nourah Bint Abdulrahman University provides two separate undergraduate programs in audiology and speech-language pathology for female students, and Dar Al-Hekmah University offers undergraduate and graduate programs in speech-language pathology for female students.

4. INTERDISCIPLINARY NATURE OF SPEECH-LANGUAGE PATHOLOGY AND AUDIOLOGY

Speech-language pathologists provide a wide range of services, most importantly on an individual basis. They also support individuals, families, support groups, and provide information for the general public on communication disorders. Their work involves prevention, assessment, diagnosis, and treatment of speech, language, social communication, cognitive-communication, and swallowing disorders in all age groups of patients. Speech-Language Pathologists also provide services with initial screening for communication and swallowing disorders and continue with assessment and diagnosis, consultation for the provision of advice regarding management, intervention, and treatment, and providing counselling and other follow up services for these disorders. The services provided by them can be listed as follows:

1) Voice – disorders of pitch such as high pitch, low pitch, puberphonia, androphonia - disorders of loudness such as aphonia, soft voice, loud voice - quality disorders such as hoarseness, harshness, breathiness – dysphonia. It is demonstrated that voice therapy is highly useful.
2) Phonation and articulation – articulation and phonological disorders either functional or organic or neurological.
3) Fluency – disorders such as stuttering, cluttering, neurogenic stuttering etc.
4) Prosody – Disorders of intonation such as monotony, disorders of stress and rhythm.
5) Cognitive aspects of communication (e.g., attention, memory, problem-solving, executive functions).
6) language (phonology, morphology, syntax, semantics, and pragmatic/social aspects of communication) including comprehension and expression in oral, written, graphic, and manual modalities; language processing; preliteracy and language-based literacy skills, phonological awareness.
7) Swallowing or other upper aerodigestive functions such as infant feeding and aeromechanical events (evaluation of esophageal function is for the purpose of referral to medical professionals).
8) Sensory awareness related to communication, swallowing, or other upper aerodigestive functions.

Introduction to Speech-Language Pathology and Audiology 205

All these disorders can result from a variety of causes, such as hearing loss, mental retardation, cerebral palsy, cleft palate, stroke, brain injury, developmental delay, or emotional issues.

Therefore, it is essential for a speech-language pathologist (SLP) to collaborate with other health care professionals, several times working as part of a multidisciplinary team. For example, all disorders arising from neurological problems require the help of a neurologist; those in children require the help of a pediatrician; those with lesions in the vocal fold require the assistance of an ENT professional, phono surgeon; those with hearing require an audiologist, those with mental retardation require a psychologist; those with cleft palate require the team of SLP, dentist, plastic surgeon, psychologist. In relation to auditory processing disorders, SLPs can collaborate in the assessment and provide intervention where there is evidence of speech, language, and/or other cognitive-communication disorders. The treatment for patients with voice disorders, cleft lip and palate is interdisciplinary. The speech therapy outcome is even better when the surgical treatment is performed earlier. A team approach provides a cross-disciplinary analysis of the patient's developmental level, learning style, and interaction patterns. This results in an integrated and functional portrait of the patient's strengths and challenges. Team members will include professionals from various disciplines and family members as needed for each patient.

The SLPs can provide referrals to audiologists and others; offer information to health care professionals (including physicians, dentists, practitioners, nurses, occupational therapists, dieticians), educators, behavior consultants and parents as dictated by the individual client's needs.

Further, SLPs work in a variety of clinical and educational settings. They work in academic institutions, public and private hospitals, skilled nursing facilities, long-term acute care facilities, terminally ill, private practice and home healthcare. SLPs may also work as part of the support structure in the education system, working in both public and private schools, colleges, and universities. Some SLPs also work in community health, providing services at prisons and young offenders' institutions. They also provide expert testimony in applicable court cases. SLPs have started delivering services via video conference or tele practice.

An audiologist provides a comprehensive array of professional services related to the prevention of hearing loss and the audiologic identification, assessment, diagnosis, and treatment of persons with impairment of auditory and vestibular function.

Audiologists should understand that patients might present with physical impairment or medical and psychological conditions that may not contribute to their symptoms. Therefore, it is imperative for an audiologist to work in team with an ENT professional, a cochlear implant surgeon, neurologist, pediatrician, speech-language pathologist, and psychologist. For example, in assessing the hearing of a patient, it is essential that the external ear canal is free from active discharge, wax etc. and therefore, the role of an ENT professional is important. For surgeries the role of an ENT professional and cochlear implant surgeon is essential. It is better to assess about the hearing before and after surgery. Children and adults with hearing loss portray speech and language problems in which case a speech-language pathologist comes in to picture. Children, and adults seeking job often may not have hearing loss; but may be malingering in which case the help of a psychologist may be needed. In case of acoustic neuroma and other neurological lesions assessment by a neurologist is a must. Therefore, an audiologist should have a network of referral and consulting specialists for patients whose problems are not merely hearing but who require additional medical, psychological, or therapeutic expertise. Patients presenting with dizziness, vertigo, or imbalance may have serious medical or even life-threatening conditions. Hence, the audiologist should be able to recognize the need for appropriate referral.

Even though hearing loss is often treatable, it sometimes goes undetected in the nursing home population and in adults with cognitive impairment as this population is difficult to test, because later stages of dementia results in a lack of attending to and understanding of test instructions. Thus, an audiologist should be able to help them understand the instructions and assess them failing which they become secluded. This comes under the array of interdisciplinary service delivery.

5. Development of Instrumentation in Speech Pathology and Audiology

5.1. Instrumentation Is Speech Pathology

Primarily the human ear was the main instrument for identification of speech disorders before the electronic age.

Pa:ṇini (4th century BCE) was an ancient Sanskrit philologist, grammarian, and a revered scholar in Hinduism. He is considered the father of Indian linguistics. His text *Aṣ.ṭa:dhya:yi*, a sutra-style treatise on Sanskrit grammar, with 3,959 "verses" or rules on linguistics, syntax and semantics in "eight chapters" is the foundational text of the *Vya:karaṇa* (grammar) branch of the Ve:da:nga. Pa:ṇini's analysis of noun compounds still forms the basis of modern linguistic theories of compounding in Indian languages. Pa:ṇini's theory of morphological analysis was more advanced than any equivalent Western theory before the 20th century. His treatise is generative and descriptive, and has been compared to the *Turing machine* wherein the logical structure of any computing device has been reduced to its essentials using an idealized mathematical model.

Pa:ṇini's work became known in 19th-century Europe, where it influenced modern linguistics initially through Franz Bopp, who mainly looked at Pa:ṇini, and subsequently, a wider body of work influenced Sanskrit scholars such as Ferdinand de Saussure, Leonard Bloomfield, and Roman Jakobson. The *Shiva Sutras in Aṣ.ṭa:dhya:yi are a brief but highly organised list of phonemes.* The phonemes are organized based on place of articulation starting from back to front of the oral tract as shown in Table 10.

Bhartṛhari (5th century CE) was a Sanskrit writer to whom are ascribed two influential Sanskrit texts - the *Va:kyapadi:ya*, and the *Śatakatraya*. *Va:kyapadiiya is a text* on Sanskrit grammar and linguistic philosophy, which is a foundational text in the Indian grammatical tradition. It explains numerous theories on the word and on the sentence, including theories which are known under the name of Sphoṭa or how a human being perceives. One can think of this as the *earliest theory of speech perception.* In this work

Bhartr̥hari also discussed logical problems such as the liar paradox and a paradox of unnameability or unsignfiability which has become known as Bhartr̥hari's paradox. *Śatakatraya is* a work of Sanskrit poetry, comprising three collections of about 100 stanzas each.

Table 10. Organization of phonemes in Sanskrit

	Velar	Palatal	retroflex	Dental	Bilabial	Velar-palatal	Bilabial	Velar-labial
Vowels	a, a:	i, i:	r,r:	lr₀, lr₀:	u, u:	e, ai	o	au

Place of articulation	Stop consonants/ affricates				Nasal continuants	Semivowels	Fricatives	
	Unvoiced		Voiced				Unvoiced	Voiced
Glottal								h
Velar	k	kh	g	gh	n·			
Palatal	c	ch	j	jh	n~		s~	
retroflex	t.	th	d.	dh	n.		s.	
Dental	t	th	d	dh	n		s	
Bilabial	p	ph	b	bh	m			
Palatal-Velar						y		
Retroflex-Velar						r		
Dental –Velar						l		
Bilabial - Velar						v		

5.1.1. A Psychophysicist

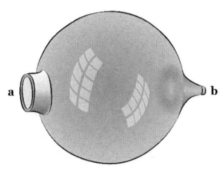

Source: https://people.seas.harvard.edu/~jones/cscie129/nu_lectures/lecture3%20/ho_helmholtz/ho_helmholtz.html.

Figure 89. Helmholtz resonator.

Herman Ludwig Ferdinand von Helmholtz (1821-1894) studied mathematics, physics and medicine and contributed to mathematics, mechanics, physiology, optics, acoustics, and electricity. Completing his study of medicine at the University of Berlin and working as a surgeon in the army, he became a professor at Konigsberg, and then at Bonn, and finally in Heidelberg and Berlin. He studied the physiology and sensation of hearing in respect of pure and complex tones. Helmholtz was the pioneer in developing the mathematics of resonance. He discovered that different sounds could be produced when one blows across the open necks of bottles with varying amounts of water in them. He could produce sounds that resembled vowels /u/, and /o/. He used hollow glass globes with two openings, known as Helmholtz resonators, and developed a technique to analyze the frequency components of complex tones. He was thus able to identify the fundamental frequency and harmonics of a human voice and the major resonant frequencies of a vocal tract much before the invention of electronic devices to analyze sounds. He held tuning forks of different frequencies in front of his mouth and those of others and asked them to shape their vocal tracts for a particular vowel. By doing so he found that different vocal tract shapes produced different resonant frequencies (formants) and determined that they were the absolute resonant frequencies of the vowel. In 1863, he published his great work on acoustics of speech and harmonic theory, *On the Sensations of Tone as a Physio local Basis for the Theory of Music*. Helmholtz is considered as the pioneer of speech acoustics. Figure 89 shows a Helmholtz resonator.

5.1.2. A Phonetician and Linguist

Henry Sweet (1845-1912), graduated from Balliol College at Oxford and was a teacher of English pronunciation. He served as a model for George Bernard Shaw's Henry Higgins in the play Pygmalion which later was adopted as My Fair Lady. Influenced by the German school of philosophy and work on phonetics in India, Sweet wrote his adaptation of Visible speech, which he called *Broad Romic*. Broad Romic is a kind of algebraic notation, each letter representing a group of similar sounds. His transcription system was a precursor of the International Phonetic Alphabet. He published the *Handbook of Phonetics* in 1877, *A History of English Sounds* in 1874, and *A Primer of Phonetics* which contained detailed articulatory descriptions of speech sounds.

5.1.3. A Speech Pathologist

Alexander Graham Bell (1847-1922), the world-renowned inventor of *telephone* was born in Edinburgh to Alexander Melville Bell, who was a speech teacher and elocutionist. Alexander Melville Bell developed *Visible Speech*, which is a system of symbols representing articulation of each speech sound. The system is composed of symbols and shows the position and movement of the throat, tongue, and lips as they produce the sounds of language, and it is a type of phonetic notation. The system was used to aid the deaf in learning to speak. In 1864 Melville promoted his first works on Visible Speech, to help the deaf both learn and improve upon their speech To help promote the language, Bell created two written short forms using his system of 29 modifiers and tones, 52 consonants, 36 vowels and a dozen diphthongs which were named World English, and was similar to the International Phonetic Alphabet, and Line Writing, used as a shorthand form for stenographers (Figure 90).

Alexander Graham Bell spent much of his time instructing teachers on the use of visible speech. He became a powerful advocate of visible speech and oralism in United States. He could pursue his mission by the money earned by the sale of patent of the telephone and Volta Laboratory patents. Unaware that he was repeating experiments of Helmholtz, Bell discovered resonances of the vocal tract cavities by snapping his finger against his throat and checking while assuming various vocal tract shapes. He also repeated experiments with tuning forks. He married Mabel Hubbard, who was deaf. "Alexander Graham Bell later devised another system of visual cues that also came to be known as visible speech. This system did not use symbols written on paper to teach deaf people how to pronounce words. Instead, Graham Bell's system, developed at his Volta Laboratory in Washington, D.C., involved the use of a spectrograph, a device that makes "visible records of the frequency, intensity, and time analysis of short samples of speech." The spectrograph translated sounds into readable patterns via a

Introduction to Speech-Language Pathology and Audiology 211

photographic process. This system was based on the idea that the eye should be able to read patterns of vocalizations in much the same way that the ear translates these vocalizations into meaning. Modern implementations of Bell's idea display sound spectra in real time and are used in phonology, speech therapy and computer speech recognition."

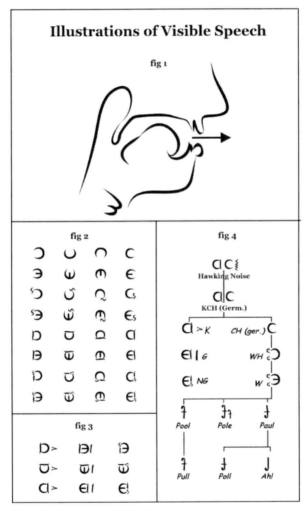

Source: https://en.wikipedia.org/wiki/Visible_Speech.

Figure 90. Visible speech.

5.1.4. A Physiologic Psychologist

In the meantime, *Raymond Herbert Stetson* (1872-1950), a doctorate from Harvard University, devoted much of his carrier to develop methods of measuring movement of respiratory mechanism and the articulators in speech production. In early 1920's he visited L'Abbe Rousselot in France who developed Kymograph (Figure 91) and on returning to USA he tried to advance the work of Rousselot's work with *Kymograph and Palatograph*. He studied the acoustic and physiologic nature of vowels and consonants. His best-known research is on the *nature of the syllable with regard to production and its structure*. His research gave rise to many other important instrumental advances. He is considered as one of the most important researchers who provided a modern scientific basis for the study of speech production.

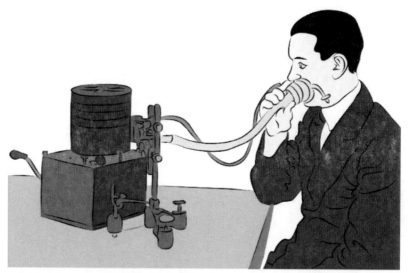

Source: https://www.english.upenn.edu/sites/www.english.upenn.edu/files/Mills-Mara_Deaf-Jam-Inscription-Reproduction-Information.pdf.

Figure 91. The first Kymograph.

Introduction to Speech-Language Pathology and Audiology 213

5.1.5. An Electrical Engineer

Homer Dudley (1896-1987) was a pioneer in speech synthesis making machines that could produce speech like sounds. The *Voder*, invented by him, in 1937 and 1938 at Bell Laboratories, the engineering laboratory of Western Electric, was the first electrical synthesizer. Earlier the *Vocoder* was to filter speech in to ten bands so that information could be transmitted over narrower bandwidths. After transmission, the channel information, along with a noise circuit for consonant sounds and a buzz circuit for phonation, was used to synthesize speech. The Vocoder was demonstrated at the tercentennial celebration at Harward and led to the celebrated talking machine, the Voder, a Voice Operated Demonstrator (Figure 92). This was shown at the 1939 and 1940 World Fair.

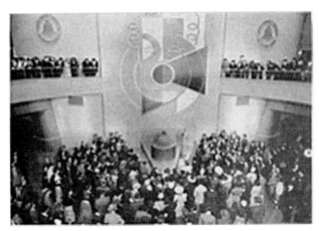

Source: https://en.wikipedia.org/wiki/Voder.

Figure 92. Voder demonstration at the World Fair, New York.

During the war time, the Russians invented the Spectrogram to identify speech and speaker. Alexander Graham Bell, a descendent from a number of phoneticians, elocutionists, speech correctionists and a teacher of hard of hearing came to America via Canada from Scotland. He founded the Bell Telephone Laboratories to provide ways to hard of hearing to learn to speak. The first device called Sonagraph came into existence in the 1930s. The Sonagraph produced 3-D patterns of phonemes which were used as visual feedback in teaching persons with hearing impairment. It provides a time-frequency-amplitude graph or a sound wave analyzer. X-axis depicts time, y-axis frequency and Z-axis (darkness) the amplitude. A moving filter swept the frequency range of a speech segment of approximately 2.5 sec duration in a narrow band (filter band width of 45 Hz) or a wide band (filter band width of 300 Hz).

In the 1940's *Ralph Potter and his colleagues*, at Bel Laboratories developed the *sound spectrograph* (Figure 93) which analyzed the frequencies of speech sounds. Potter conceived the reverse of the sound spectrograph as a machine which could convert the visible patters to sounds. At Haskins Laboratories, *Franklin Cooper* (1908-1999), a Physicist, understood that such a *Pattern Play Back* (Figure 94) would be a powerful machine for the study of speech perception. The Pattern Play Back was capable of converting spectrograms and hand painted copies of spectrograms to intelligible speech. *Alvin Liberman*, a Psychologist, who succeeded Cooper, used Pattern Play Back to vary the acoustic parameters of speech systematically to understand the cues used for speech perception. *Pierre Delattre*, a French Linguist, helped to develop the rules for painting synthetic patterns without referring to the actual spectrograms, and composed a piece of synthetic music which he called *Scotch Plaid*. Cooper, Liberman, and Delatrre produced most of the early work in speech perception.

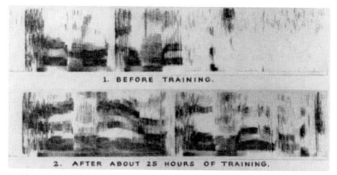

Source: https://www.english.upenn.edu/sites/www.english.upenn.edu/files/Mills-Mara_Deaf-Jam-Inscription-Reproduction-Information.pdf.

Figure 93. The sound spectrograph.

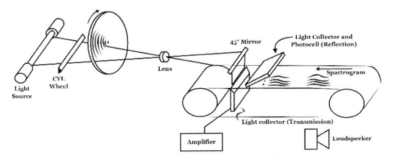

Source: http://www.haskins.yale.edu/featured/patplay.html.

Figure 94. The Pattern Play Back.

The invention of computer led to their use in the field of speech pathology. It was used to measure fundamental frequency, its range, to obtain spectrograms, to develop software that could measure the airflow and other measures of the respiratory system and to certain extent synthesize speech. Further to this, Electromyography was used to measure the movements of muscles. *Electromyography (EMG)* (Figure 95) is an electrodiagnostic medicine technique for evaluating and recording the electrical activity produced by skeletal muscles. It detects the electric potential generated by muscle cells when these cells are electrically or neurologically activated. The signals can be analyzed to detect medical abnormalities, activation level, or to analyze the biomechanics of human or animal movement.

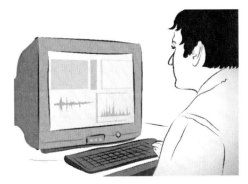

Source: https://en.wikipedia.org/wiki/Electromyography.

Figure 95. An Electromyograph.

Manometers, Spirometers and Pneumotachograph were used for respiratory analysis. *Pressure measurement* is the analysis of an applied force by a fluid (liquid or gas) on a surface. It is measured in units of force per unit of surface area. Several techniques were developed for the measurement of pressure and vacuum. Instruments used to measure, and display pressure are called pressure gauges or vacuum gauges. A *manometer* (Figure 96) is an example of pressure gauge. It uses a column of liquid to both measure and indicates pressure.

A *spirometer* is an apparatus that measures the volume of air inspired and expired by the lungs. Various types of spirometers (pressure transducers, ultrasonic, water gauge) are used for a number of different methods for measurement.

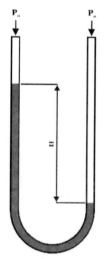

Source: https://en.wikipedia.org/wiki/Pressure_measurement.

Figure 96. A Manometer.

Laryngeal activities were recorded by laryngoscope (Figure 97), developed in 1854 by *Manual Patricia Rodriguez Garcia*, a Spanish singing teacher, high speed motion pictures initially, and then a stroboscope, a laryngoscope, a fiberoptic endoscope. Other non-invasive techniques include electroglottogram.

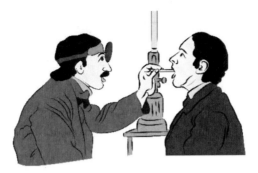

Manual Garcia using his laryngoscope

Source: http://www.enttoday.org/article/history-of-the-laryngoscope/.

Figure 97. A laryngeal mirror used by Manuel Garcia.

The *electroglottograph*, or *EGG* (Figure 98), sometimes referred to as a laryngograph was founded by *Fourcin in* 1971. It is a device used for the non-invasive measurement of the degree of contact between the vibrating vocal folds during voice production. Two electrodes are placed on the surface of the neck and a small electrical current is passed between them. The EGG records variations in the transverse electrical impedance of the larynx and nearby tissues. This electrical impedance will vary slightly with the area of contact between the moist vocal folds during vibrations. Early commercially available EGG units were compared quite thoroughly by Baken.

Articulatory analysis was carried out with x-ray photography, the ultrasound, palatography, electropalatography, and EMMA. *Electropalatography* (EPG) (Figure 99) is a technique used to monitor contacts between the tongue and hard palate, particularly during articulation and speech. A custom-made artificial palate is molded to fit against a speaker's hard palate. The artificial palate contains electrodes exposed to the lingual surface. When contact occurs between the tongue surface and any of the electrodes, electrical signals are sent to an external processing unit. EPG was originally conceptualized and developed as a tool for phonetics research to improve upon traditional palatography. Both military and academic language researchers used early electropalatography tools to get information regarding tongue-to-palate contact.

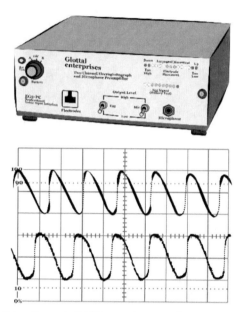

Source; https://en.wikipedia.org/wiki/Electroglottograph.

Figure 98. An Electroglottograph and the EGG signal (Glottal enterprises).

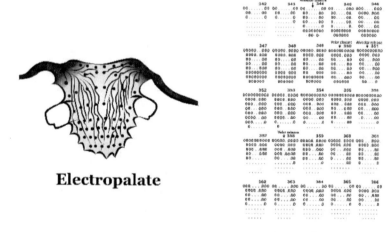

Source: https://en.wikipedia.org/wiki/Electropalatography.

Figure 99. Electropalate and EPG.

Visualization of the activity of brain is very important in the understanding of speech production and perception. The Event Related Potentials, Positron Emission Tomography, and magnetic imaging (fMRI) have been important instruments used towards this. An *event-related potential (ERP)* (Figure 100) is the measured brain response as a result of a specific sensory, cognitive, or motor event. It is a non-invasive means of evaluating brain functioning. *Hans Berger*, in 1924, showed that one could measure the electrical activity of the human brain by placing electrodes on the scalp and amplifying the signal using *electroencephalogram*. Further the changes in voltage can be plotted over a period of time. In 1935–1936, *Pauline and Hallowell Davis* recorded the first known ERPs on awake humans and their findings were published a few years later, in 1939. *Sutton, Braren, Zubin & John* (1965) made advancement with the discovery of the P3 component. ERPs are one of the most widely used methods in cognitive neuroscience research to investigate the physiological correlates of sensory, perceptual and cognitive activity associated with processing information.

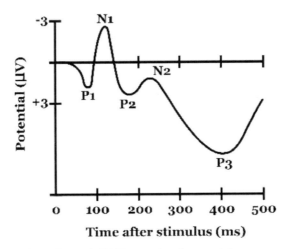

Source: https://en.wikipedia.org/wiki/Event-related_potential.

Figure 100. ERP showing P1, N1, P2, and N2.

5.2. Development of Instrumentation in Audiology

It is impossible and not required here to write chapters on instrumentation in Audiology. Rather, the section will briefly introduce the development of instrumentation in Audiology.

Initially, the requirement was to produce sounds that could repeat, control intensity, transmit the sound, record the response of the subject and interpret it. Various devices that produced sounds with control in intensity were used in the beginning. Some of them included clock-like device, a tripped hammer to strike a metal rod, a tuning fork. Perhaps the first measurement device for testing hearing was described by Wolke (1802). The device had a wooden board placed upright and a drumstick, which could be dropped onto the board from various heights, was attached to it. The height could be read from a related scale. Wolke tested the usefulness of this "*acuity meter*" on deaf mutes. Variations of this were available until the end of the 19th century (Silman & Emmer, 2012).

Induction coil was developed between 1836 to 1860 and telephone in the year 1876. Following these, a variety of audiometers was invented all over the world and was known as induction-coil audiometers. In 1899, *Carl E. Seashore* Professor of Psychology at University of Iowa, United States, introduced the *audiometer* as an instrument to measure the "keenness of hearing." This instrument operated on a battery and presented a tone or a click and had an attenuator set in a scale of 40 steps. This became the basis of the audiometers later manufactured by *Western Electric*.

The concept of plotting frequency versus sensitivity (amplitude), a plot of human hearing sensitivity was envisaged by German physicist Max Wien in 1903. Two groups of researchers —Schaefer and Gruschke, Griessmann and Schwarzkopf -, in 1919, demonstrated two vacuum tube instruments designed to test hearing acuity before the Berlin Otological Society. However, neither of the two devices was developed commercially for some time; but the second was to be manufactured under the name *Otaudion*.

In the year 1922, otolaryngologist *Dr. Edmund P. Fowler,* and *physicists Dr. Harvey Fletcher and Robert Wegel* of Western Electric Co. were the first to plot frequency at octave intervals along the abscissa and intensity

Introduction to Speech-Language Pathology and Audiology 221

downward along the ordinate as a degree of hearing loss and termed the graph as *audiogram*. With technological advances bone conduction testing was also included by 1928. An audiometer is an electronic instrument to test human hearing. As on date, audiometers with various types of test stimuli, varieties of frequency range, manual Vs. automatic, diagnostic Vs. screening, and with different number of channels are available in the market.

The term immittance was invented by Bode (1945). Immittance is a concept combining the impedance and admittance of a system or circuit. Tympanometry is sometimes referred to as immittance testing. *Tympanometry* is used to test the condition of the middle ear, mobility of the tympanic membrane, and the conduction of middle ear bones by creating variations of air pressure in the ear canal.

The *auditory brainstem response (ABR)* is an auditory evoked potential extracted from ongoing electrical activity in the brain and recorded via electrodes placed on the scalp. *Sohmer and Feinmesser*, in 1967, were the first to publish ABRs recorded with surface electrodes in humans and this showed that cochlear potentials could be obtained non-invasively. The measured recording has a series of six to seven vertex positive waves. Waves I through V are usually evaluated. *Jewett and Williston* labelled these waves with Roman numerals which occur in the first 10 milliseconds after onset of an auditory stimulus. The ABR is considered an *exogenous response* because it is dependent upon external factors.

Georg von Békésy (1899-1972), a Hungarian biophysicist born in Budapest was awarded the Nobel Prize in Physiology or Medicine for his research on the function of the cochlea in the mammalian hearing organ in the year 1961. He measured the acoustic impedance of the ear with varying ear canal air pressures. Knut Terkildsen, in 1964, was the first to use the term *tympanometry* to describe the effect of ear canal pressure on impedance.

David Kemp, in 1978, reported that sound energy produced by the ear could be detected in the ear canal. An *otoacoustic emission (OAE)* is a sound which is generated from within the inner ear. The first commercial system for detecting and measuring OAEs was developed in 1988.

A *hearing aid* is a device designed to improve hearing. The first hearing aids were ear trumpets that were created in the 17th century. A movement towards modern hearing aids began with the invention of the telephone. The first electric hearing aid, the *akouphone*, was created around 1895 by Miller Reese Hutchison. The invention of the carbon microphone, transmitters, digital signal processing chip, and the development of computer technology helped transform the hearing aid and by the late 20th century, digital hearing aids were commercially available.

A *cochlear implant* is a surgically implanted electronic device that provides a sense of sound to a person who is hard of hearing in both ears. Cochlear implants bypass the normal hearing process; they have a sound processor that resides on the outside of the skin and generally worn behind the ear which contains microphones, electronics, battery, and a coil that transmits a signal to the implant. The implant has a coil to receive signals, and an array of electrodes which is surgically placed into the cochlea, and can stimulate the cochlear nerve. The first cochlear implant was invented by Dr. William House, in 1961. Blair Simmons and Robert J. White, in the year 1964, implanted a six channel electrode in a patient's cochlea at Stanford University. The modern multichannel cochlear implant was independently developed and commercialized by Graeme Clark from Australia. Ingeborg Hochmair and Erwin Hochmair, with the Hochmairs' first implanted in a person in 1977 and Clark's in 1978.

5.3. Scope of Practice in Speech-Language Pathology and Audiology

This document is taken from the Indian Speech & Hearing Association website (http://www.ishaindia.org.in/pdf/Scope_of_Practice.pdf).

Development of a *Scope of Practice* document was initiated and finalized in 2015. This document describes the range of interests, capabilities and professional activities of speech-language pathologists and audiologists. Certification will be by the Rehabilitation Council of India. The scope of practice is consistent with the principles of the International Classification of functioning disability and Health (ICF) recommended by the World Health Organization (WHO, 2001) and guidelines of the United

Introduction to Speech-Language Pathology and Audiology 223

Nations convention on Rights of Persons with disabilities (United Nation, 2006).

The document is intended to

a) define areas of practice for Speech-Language Pathologists and Audiologists functioning independently or as a member of a multidisciplinary team,

b) serve as a resource for health care professionals, regulatory bodies, Government agencies, educators, consumers, and general public and any other stake holders,

c) serve as a reference on issues relating to service delivery, man power development, employment, insurance, legislation, consumer education, regulatory action, professional licensure, planning, and inter-professional relations,

d) provide guidance for the development of curricula for man power training programs in Speech-Language Pathologists and Audiology, and

e) to support and guide Speech-Language Pathologists and Audiologists in their educational preparation, professional development and research activities.

The undergraduate programme in India has both Speech-Language Pathology and Audiology and combined and bifurcated programs are available at the master's level. Speech-Language Pathologists and Audiologists provide their services to all individuals across the age span from birth through adulthood, irrespective of languages, religions and beliefs, and ethnic, cultural, and socio-economic backgrounds.

The activities described in this document are not an exhaustive list of professional responsibilities of Speech-Language Pathologists and Audiologists. As a dynamic and growing profession, the fields of Speech-Language Pathology and Audiology ought to transform over time because of the as new information acquired. Hence the Scope of Practice document will be reviewed regularly for consistency with current knowledge and practice.

It is not necessary that a Speech-Language Pathologist and Audiologist practice in all the areas described in this document. Individual professionals may limit or expand their practice based on their interest, expertise, training, and circumstances. As the list is not exhaustive, the members may also provide services not stated in this document. Speech-Language Pathologists and Audiologists are ethically bound to provide services that are consistent with the scope of their training, competence, and experience. Speech-Language Pathologists and Audiologists shall continually update and improve their knowledge and skills by attending Continuing Rehabilitation Education Programs, conventions, seminars, workshops, and other professional development programs.

5.3.1. Definition

Though a Speech-Language Pathologist and Audiologist is a part of an integrated health care system in India, they are independent in their work. Or the work of Speech-Language Pathologist and Audiologist shall not be supervised or prescribed by any other professional.

"Speech-Language Pathologist is a qualified professional who provides a comprehensive array of professional services related to the identification, diagnosis and management of persons with communication and swallowing disorders. Speech-Language Pathologists are involved in activities to promote effective communication and swallowing and prevent disorders of such processes. A Speech-Language Pathologist is a professional who engages in clinical services, prevention, advocacy, education, administration, and research in the broad areas of communication and swallowing" (http://www.ishaindia.org.in/pdf/Scope_of_Practice.pdf).

"Audiologist is a qualified professional who provides a comprehensive array of professional services related to the identification, diagnosis and management of persons with auditory (peripheral and central), balance, and related disorders, and the prevention of these impairments. They facilitate prevention through the fitting of hearing protective devices, education programs for industry and the public, hearing screening/ conservation programs, and research. Audiologists may also engage in research pertinent

to all of these domains" (http://www.ishaindia.org.in/pdf/Scope_of_ Practice.pdf).

The overall objective of the provision of Speech-Language Pathology and Audiology services is to optimize and enhance the ability of the individual to speak, communicate, and to hear. In addition, Speech-Language Pathologists and Audiologists may assist normal individuals who interact with persons with communication impairments.

The designation of Speech and hearing professionals in India should be specified as one of the following:

a) Speech-Language Pathologist
b) Audiologist
c) Speech-Language Pathologist and Audiologist
d) Audiologist and Speech-Language Pathologist
e) Speech therapist and Audiologist

The document further stipulates that

a) The words speech therapist and speech-language pathologist mean the same and can be used inter-changeably, and
b) Though personnel with a Diploma in Speech, Language and Hearing or Communication Disorders can dispense services for the needy, s/he shall do so only under the supervision of a Speech-Language Pathologist and or Audiologist with at least an undergraduate degree.

5.3.2. Educational Requirements/Qualifications

Speech-Language Pathologists and Audiologists complete an undergraduate or a master's or a doctoral degree in the field of speech, language and hearing from a recognized University from India or abroad. The master's and the doctoral programs currently include a combined program in Speech-Language Pathology and Audiology as well as specialization in Speech-Language Pathology, and Audiology.

In addition to a degree from a recognized University, the institutions/ colleges conducting programs in Speech-Language Pathology and or Audiology are recognized by the Rehabilitation Council of India (RCI). Only those with a recognized degree in the field and registered with the Rehabilitation Council of India can practice Speech-Language Pathology and or Audiology in India. RCI requires proof of continued development for the maintenance of membership in its Central Rehabilitation Register.

5.3.3. Professional Roles and Responsibilities

Speech-Language Pathologists and Audiologists provide a broad range of services to persons with speech, language, communication and hearing disorders as shown below:

5.3.4. Clinical Services: Speech-Language Pathology

5.3.4.1. Prevention and Identification

Screening for speech, orofacial and myofunctional disorders, language, cognitive communication disorders, and preferred communication modalities that may have a bearing on education, health, development or communication.

5.3.4.2. Assessment

a) Clinical or instrumental screening, identification, assessment, diagnosis, and management of
- Speech sound disorders and delays
- Language delays and disorders
- Fluency disorders
- Phonation and resonance disorders
- Neurogenic communication disorders
- Swallowing and feeding disorders
- Cognitive-communication disorders including disorders of social communication skills, attention, memory, reasoning, sequencing, problem solving and executive functions

Introduction to Speech-Language Pathology and Audiology 227

- Pre-literacy and literacy skills including phonological awareness, decoding, reading comprehension and writing.
- Communication and swallowing disorders in the context of other diagnoses or impairments including but not limited to hearing impairments, traumatic brain injury, dementia, developmental, intellectual or genetic disorders, and neurological impairments.
- Speech disorders due to structural abnormalities like laryngectomy, glossectomy, cleft palate etc.

5.3.4.3. Management and Rehabilitation

a) Management of all kinds of speech-language, communication and swallowing disorders through instrumental and/ or behavioral methods including expert advice for their medical/ surgical management.

b) Improvement of speech-language proficiency, communication effectiveness, and care and improvement of professional voice.

c) Development, assessment and selection of augmentative and alternative communication systems including unaided and aided strategies.

d) Selecting, fitting and establishing effective use of prosthetic/ adaptive devices for communication and swallowing.

e) Consultation and training for development of effective communication skills in social and other settings.

f) Counselling affected individuals, their family members, co-workers, educators, and other persons in the community regarding enhancing communication environment, acceptance, adaptation, and decision making about communication and swallowing.

g) Medico legal consultation and advice including applications in forensic science.

5.3.5. Clinical Services: Audiology

5.3.5.1. Prevention and Identification

a) Promotion of hearing health – Prevention of hearing disorders in children and adults by conducting appropriate hearing conservation and noise management programs in schools, industries, and community. This also includes selection, counselling, and monitoring, of the use of hearing protection devices such as ear muffs, ear plugs etc.

b) Supervision, implementation, and follow-up of new-born and school hearing screening programs.

5.3.5.2. Assessment

a) Clinical and/or instrumental screening, identification, assessment, and diagnosis of
- Hearing disorders involving peripheral or central pathways of hearing in persons of all ages.
- Hearing related disorders like tinnitus, hyperacusis etc.
- Hearing system related balance disorders, and
- Auditory related processing disorders.

b) The conduct and interpretation of behavioral, electroacoustic, and / or electrophysiological methods to assess hearing, auditory function, balance, and related systems.

c) Assessment of candidacy of persons with hearing loss for cochlear implants and provision of fitting, mapping, and audiologic/ educative rehabilitation to optimize device use.

d) Electro diagnostic tests for purposes of neurophysiologic intraoperative monitoring and cranial nerve assessment

5.3.5.3. Management and Rehabilitation

a) Management of hearing and hearing system-related balance disorders through instrumental and / or behavioral methods including expert advice for their medical / surgical management.

Introduction to Speech-Language Pathology and Audiology   229

b) Assessment, selection. Fitment and dispensing of all kinds of hearing assistive devices including hearing aids and (re)habilitation regimens for individuals with hearing impairment, hearing system-related disorders, tinnitus and other auditory-related disorders, Rehabilitation regimens include adult and child aural (re)habilitation, speech reading, tinnitus retraining, vestibular (re)habilitation, manual communication etc.

c) Development and implementation of an audiologic rehabilitation plan including
  - Hearing aid fitment, educating the consumer and caregivers in the use of and adjustment to hearing-related sensory aids, counselling related to psycho-social aspects of auditory dysfunction, and environmental modifications to facilitate development of receptive and expressive communication.
  - Participation in the development of an individual education program for school-age children, and provision for in-service programs for school personnel in planning educational programs for children with auditory dysfunction.
  - Selection, installation, and evaluation of large-area amplification systems.

d) Consultation with and referrals to professionals in related and / or allied field, services, agencies, and / or consumer organizations.

e) Medico legal consultation and advice including applications in forensic science.

5.3.6. Services/Functions Common to Speech-Language Pathologists and Audiologists

The following are some of the common services provided by speech-language pathologists and audiologists relating to their respective domains of specialization.

5.3.6.1. Advocacy

a) Counselling and education services to clients, families, caregivers, other professionals, and the public regarding all aspects of speech, language, communication, swallowing, hearing and auditory function.

b) Advocacy for the rights/ funding of services with hearing loss, auditory dysfunction, balance dysfunction, auditory-related disorders, communication and swallowing disorders, and populations at risk.

c) Consultation to educators as members of interdisciplinary teams about individual educational program, communication management, educational implications of communication disorders, hearing loss and auditory dysfunctions, educational programming, classroom acoustics, and large-area amplification systems for children with hearing loss and other auditory dysfunction.

d) Consultation on assessment and management of educational. Workplace and other public acoustic environments.

e) Consultation with government, industry and community agencies regarding improvements relating to legislations on disability, rights of the disabled, noise and environment etc., and implementation of environmental and occupational voice and hearing conservation program.

f) Consultation with workers compensation boards and relevant governmental bodies regarding criteria and determination of pension/ benefits for individual with hearing loss and related disorders.

g) Consultation to industry on the development of products and instrumentation relating to identification and assessment of speech, language, communication, swallowing, hearing, balance, and auditory functions.

h) Consultation to individuals and private agencies and governmental bodies, or as an expert witness regarding legal interpretations of findings and legislations relating to all dimensions of speech, language and hearing.

Introduction to Speech-Language Pathology and Audiology 231

5.3.6.2. Research and Man Power Development

Speech-Language Pathologists and Audiologists are involved in conducting basic and applied research related to normal processes and disorders of hearing, balance, communication, swallowing, and other related aspects. Speech-Language Pathologists and Audiologists are involved in the design and conduct of basic and applied research to increase that knowledge base, to develop new develops and programs, and to determine the efficacy, effectiveness, and efficiency of assessment and treatment paradigms: disseminate research findings to other professionals and to the public in the relevant fields.

Speech-Language Pathologists and Audiologists serve as educators in University and/or college education and training programs related to communication sciences and disorders and swallowing as well as hearing science and disorders. Some of the activities are as follows:

- Imparting educational different levels – certificate, diploma, degree, master's and doctoral – in the broad areas of speech-language pathology and audiology,
- Framing syllabi, curricula, clinical modules and policies related to training of professionals in speech-language pathology and audiology, and related inter/ trans disciplinary fields,
- Developing policies, operational procedures, professional standard and quality improvement programs in the fields of speech-language pathology and audiology, and
- Public education and in-service training to families, caregivers, and other professionals.

5.3.6.3. Administration

- Development, administration and management of clinical programs.
- Administering and managing academic institutions running certificate, diploma and degree programs at graduate, post-graduate, and doctoral levels in the field of speech-language pathology and audiology.

- Administration in government (state and central) and non-governmental agencies and institutions related to disability in general and speech-language pathology and/ or audiology in particular as per the directions of the agencies and institutions.

5.3.6.4. Others

a) Consultation with, and referrals to, professionals in related and / or allied fields, services, agencies, and / or consumer organizations.
b) Medico-legal consultation and advice including applications in forensic science.
c) Quantification and certification of disability relating to all kinds of speech, language, hearing, communication, and related disorders.
d) Screening, assessment, management and rehabilitation can be through direct (face to face) or tele-mode.

5.3.6.5. Practice Settings

Speech-language pathologists and audiologists work in a variety of settings including but not limited to:

- Health care settings (including hospitals, clinics, nursing homes, medical rehabilitation centers, mental health facilities),
- Regular and special schools,
- Early intervention programs/ multidisciplinary rehabilitation centers,
- Industrial settings,
- Hearing aid and cochlear implant manufacturers,
- Manufacturers of devices/prothesis for individuals with communication and swallowing disorders,
- Universities/colleges and their clinics,
- Professional associations,
- State and central government agencies and institutions,
- Research centers, and
- Private practice settings.

Introduction to Speech-Language Pathology and Audiology 233

(http://www.ishaindia.org.in/pdf/Scope_of_Practice.pdf)

The audiologist is an integral part of the team within the school system that manages students with hearing impairments and students with central auditory processing disorders. The audiologist participates in the development of Individual Family Service Plans (IFSPs) and Individualized Educational Programs (IEPs), serves as a consultant in matters pertaining to classroom acoustics, assistive listening systems, hearing aids, communication, and psycho-social effects of hearing loss, and maintains both classroom assistive systems as well as students' personal hearing aids. The audiologist administers hearing screening programs in schools and trains and supervises non-audiologists performing hearing screening in the educational setting.

5.3.6.6. Hearing Conservation

The audiologist designs, implements and coordinates industrial and community hearing conservation programs. This includes identification and amelioration of noise-hazardous conditions, identification of hearing loss, recommendation and counselling on use of hearing protection, employee education, and the training and supervision of non-audiologists performing hearing screening in the industrial setting.

5.3.6.7. Intraoperative Neurophysiologic Monitoring

Audiologists administer and interpret electrophysiologic measurements of neural function including, but not limited to, sensory and motor evoked potentials, tests of nerve conduction velocity, and electromyography. These measurements are used in differential diagnosis, pre- and postoperative evaluation of neural function, and neurophysiologic intraoperative monitoring of central nervous system, spinal cord, and cranial nerve function.

5.3.6.8. Research

Audiologists design, implement, analyze and interpret the results of research related to auditory and balance systems.

5.3.6.9. Additional Expertise

Some audiologists, by virtue of education, experience and personal choice choose to specialize in an area of practice not otherwise defined in this document. Nothing in this document shall be construed to limit individual freedom of choice in this regard provided that the activity is consistent with the American Academy of Audiology Code of Ethics.

This document will be reviewed, revised, and updated periodically in order to reflect changing clinical demands of audiologists and in order to keep pace with the changing scope of practice reflected by these changes and innovations in this specialty.

CONCLUSION

The last chapter covered historical aspects of the field of speech-language pathology, and audiology, development of speech and language pathology and audiology both in Indian and global context, development of instrumentation in Speech Pathology both Indian and western origin and development of instrumentation in Audiology. Later scope of Practice in Speech-Language Pathology and Audiology was addressed.

With this, the book introduced the fields of Speech-Language Pathology & Audiology by covering speech production, hearing mechanism, basic concepts required to further learn Speech- Language Pathology and Audiology and lastly the historical aspects. It is hoped that the book will imbibe the reader for understanding, generating interest & ideas by the simple illustration, further reading, questioning and communicating with it.

REFERENCES

Aesop. 6th Century B C. Retrieved from http://www.acsu.buffalo. edu/~duchan/new_history/ancient_history/major_players.html. Accessed January 20.

Introduction to Speech-Language Pathology and Audiology 235

Alanazi, A. A. 2017. "Audiology and speech-language pathology practice in Saudi Arabia." *Int J Health Sci (Qassim).*, 11(5):43-55.

Albertus Magnus. 1193 – 1282. Retrieved from http://www.acsu.buffalo. edu/~duchan/new_history/middle_ages/major_players.html. Accessed January 20.

Anderson, Douglas. 1997. *The enlightenment of Benjamin Franklin*, Baltimore: John Hopkins University Press.

Anon. 1927. Cited in Judy Duchans *A History of Speech Language Pathology.* 19th Century. Retrieved from http://www.acsu.buffalo.edu/ ~duchan/new_history/enlightenment/sheridan.html. Accessed January 20.

Aristotle. 384 – 322 BCE. Retrieved from https://www.acsu.buffalo. edu/~duchan/new_history/ancient_history/greece.html. Accessed January 20.

Baken, R. J., and Orlikoff, R. F. 2000. *Clinical Measurement of Speech and Voice.* (2nd Ed.).San Diago: Singular Publishing Co.

Ball, M. J., and Code, C. (Eds.). 1997. *Instrumental Clinical Phonetics*, London: Whurr Publications.

Bell, Alexander Melville. 1867. *Visible Speech: The Science of Universal Alphabetics*, London: Simkin, Marshall & Co.

Benzie, W. 1972. *The Dublin orator: Thomas Sheridan's influence on eighteenth century rhetoric and belles letters.* UK: University of Leeds.

Bhate, S., and Kak, S. 1993. "Panini and Computer Science." *Annals of the Bhandarkar Oriental Research Institute*, Vol. 72, 79–94.

Blanton, S. 1882 – 1966. Retrieved from http://www.acsu.buffalo. edu/~duchan/history_subpages/smileyblanton.html. Accessed January 20.

Bloomfield, L. 1939. "Linguistic aspects of science." *International Encyclopedia of Unified Science, 1, 4,* viii + 59.

Bode, H. W. 1945. *Network Analysis and Feedback Amplifier Design.* Princeton: Van Nostrand Co Inc.

Caelius Aurelianus. 5th Century A D. Retrieved from http://www.acsu.buffalo.edu/~duchan/new_history/ancient_history/major_players.html. Accessed January 20.

Caraka. pre-2nd Century. 1867. *Caraka samhita*, Bombay: Nirnaya Sagara Press. 3-8-61.

Cardona, George. 1997. 1976. *Pāṇini: A Survey of Research, Motilal Banarsidass, ISBN 978-81-208-1494-3.*

Carl Emil Seashore. 1866-1949. Retrieved from http://www.acsu.buffalo.edu/~duchan/new_history/hist19c/subpages/seashore.html. Accessed January 20.

Ceponiene, R., Cummings, A., Wulfeck, B., Ballantyne, A., and Townsend, J. 2009. "Spectral vs. temporal auditory processing in specific language impairment: A developmental ERP study." *Brain & Language.* 110 (3): 107–20. PMC 2731814. PMID 19457549. doi:10.1016/j.bandl.2009.04.003.

Clark, G. 1977. Cited in A. Mudry, & Mara Mills.2013. "The early history of the cochlear implant: a retrospective." *JAMA otolaryngology - head & neck surgery.* 139 (5): 446–53.

Claudius. 10 B C – 54 A D. Retrieved from http://www.acsu.buffalo.edu/~duchan/new_history/ancient_history/major_players.html. Accessed January 20.

Coles, M. G. H. and Rugg, M. D. 1995. "Event-related brain potentials: An introduction. In *Electrophysiology of mind: Event-related brain potentials and cognition*, edited by M. D. Rugg, and M. G. H. Coles. Oxford psychology series, No. 25. New York: Oxford University Press. 1–26.

Comstock, A. 1795-1864. Retrieved from http://www.acsu.buffalo.edu/~duchan/new_history/hist19c/subpages/comstock.html. Accessed January 20.

Cooper, F. S., Delattre, P. C., Liberman, A. M., Borst, J. M., and Gerstman, L. J. 1952. "Some Experiments on the Perception of Synthetic Speech Sounds." *J. Acoust. Soc. Amer.,* 24, 597.

Cooper, F. S., Liberman, A. M., and Borst, J. M. 1951. "The interconversion of audible and visible patterns as a basis for research in the perception

Introduction to Speech-Language Pathology and Audiology 237

of speech." *Proceedings of the National Academy of Sciences*, 1951, 37,318-325.

Cremin, L. 1970. *American education: The colonial experience*, 1607-1783. New York: Harper and Row.

Damasio, A. 1994. *Descartes' error*. New York: G.P. Putnam's Sons.

Darwin, E. 1731-1802. https://www.mnsu.edu/comdis/kuster/history/bgoldberg.html. Accessed January 20.

Dennis H. Klatt. 1987. "Review of text-to-speech conversion for English." *J. Acoust. Soc. Amer.* 82: 737 - 793.

Dr. Paul Broca. *Science.* 1 (8): 93. 21 August 1880. doi:10.1126/science.os-1.9.93. JSTOR 2900242. Accessed January 20.

Duchan, J. 2010. "John Thelwall's elocutionary practices" *Romanticism*, 16, 2, 191-196.

Duchan, J. Retrieved from http://www.acsu.buffalo.edu/~duchan/history.html. Accessed January 20.

Eustacia. 6th Century A D. Retrieved from http://www.acsu.buffalo.edu/~duchan/new_history/middle_ages/major_players.html. Accessed January 20.

Finger, S., and Buckingham, H. 1994. Alexander Crichton. 1763 – 1856. "Disorders of fluent speech and associationist theory." *Archives of Neurology*, 51, 5, 498-503.

Floyd Summer Muckey. 1858 – 1930. Retrieved from http://www.acsu.buffalo.edu/~duchan/new_history/hist19c/subpages/muckey.html. Accessed January 20.

Fourcin, A., and Abberton, E. 1972. "First applications of a new laryngograph." *Volta Review*, 69, 507-518 {reprinted from Med. & Biol. Illustration 21, (1971), 172-182}.

Fowler, E. P., Fletcher, H., and Wegel, R. 1922. Retrieved from https://en.wikipedia.org/wiki/Audiometry. Accessed January 20.

Galambos, Robert. 2010. Hallowell Davis: 1896—1992, *National Academy of Science.* Accessed January 20.

García, Manuel. 1855. "Observations on the Human Voice." *Proceedings of the Royal Society of London. 7: 399–410. doi:10.1098/rspl. 1854.0094. JSTOR 111815.*

238   *S. R. Savithri*

Garey L. J. 2006. *Brodmann's Localisation in the Cerebral Cortex*. New York: Springer. ISBN 978-0387-26917-7.

Gelfand, S. A. 2009. *Essentials of Audiology* (3rd Ed.). New York: Thieme Medical Publishers, Inc.

Geschwind, D. H. 2009. Cited in Konopka, G., Bomar, J. M., Winden, K, Coppola, G., Jonsson, Z. O., Gao, F., Peng, S, Preuss, T., Wohlschlege, J. A., and Geschwind, D. H. 2009. "Human-specific transcriptional regulation of CNS development genes by FOXP2. "*Nature*, Vol. 462|12.

Gesner, J. A. P. 1770. Retrieved from http://www.acsu.buffalo.edu/~duchan/history.html.Graeme Clark from Australia. Accessed January 20.

Gesner, J. A. P. 1770. Retrieved from http://www.acsu.buffalo.edu/~duchan/history.html. Accessed January 20.

Glass, Bentley 1959. *Forerunners of Darwin*. Baltimore, MD: Johns Hopkins University Press. p. iv. ISBN 978-0-8018-0222-5.

Glorig, A. 1973. "Georg von Békésy 1899–1972." *Audiology, 12 (5), 540–1, doi:10.3109/00206097309071667, PMID 4582926.*

Goddard, P. E. 1905. *Mechanical Aids to the Study and Recording of Language*. Proc. of the American Anthroplogical Association. Vol. 7, No. 4, 613-619. Caliornia: Wiley.

Goggin, J., Thompson, C., Strube, G., and Simental, L. 1991. "The role of language familiarity in voice identification." *Memory Cogn.*, 19, 448-458.

Greene, E. B. 1914. "The Anglican outlook on the American Colonies in the early 18th Century." *American Historical Review, XX*, 64-85.

Haas, L. F. 2003. "Hans Berger 1873-1941. Richard Caton 1842-1926. and electroencephalography." *Journal of Neurology, Neurosurgery & Psychiatry*. 74 (1): 9. doi:10.1136/jnnp.74.1.9. PMC 1738204. PMID 12486257.

Heinrich Rudolf Hertz. 1857 – 1894. *International Electrotechnical commission History*. Iec.ch.

Henry Pieron. 1956. "Geza Revesz: 1878-1955." in: *The American Journal of Psychology*, Vol. 69, No. 1. 139-141.

Hergenhahn, B. R. 2001. *An introduction to the history of psychology.* Belmont, CA: Wadsworth/Thomson Learning.

Hermann Ludwig Ferdinand von Helmholtz. 1896. *On the sensation of tone: Theory of Music* (3rd Ed). London: Longmans, Green and Co.

Herzberger, Hans and Radhika Herzberger. 1981. "Bhartrhari's Paradox." *Journal of Indian Philosophy 9: 1-17* (slightly revised version of "Bhartrhari's Paradox" in Studies in Indian Philosophy. A memorial volume in honour of pandit Sukhlalji Sanghvi. (L.D. Series 84.) Gen. ed. Dalsukh Malvania et al. Ahmedabad, 1981).

Hoff, H.E., Guillemin, R., and Geddes, L. 1954. "An 18th century scientist's observations on his own aphasia." *Bulletin of the History of Medicine, 32,* 446–450.

House, W. F. 1976. "Cochlear implants." *Ann Otol Rhinol Laryngol.,* 85 (3, pt 2):(suppl 27).

http://rehabcouncil.nic.in. Accessed January 20.

http://www.acsu.buffalo.edu/~duchan/history_summary.html. Accessed January 20.

http://www.acsu.buffalo.edu/~duchan/new_history/hist19c/intro.html. Accessed January 20.

http://www.haskins.yale.edu/featured/patplay.html. Accessed January 20.

http://www.ishaindia.org.in/aboutus.html. Accessed January 20.

http://www.ishaindia.org.in/pdf/Scope_of_Practice.pdf. Accessed January 20.

https://en.wikipedia.org/wiki/Homer_Dudley. Accessed January 20.

https://en.wikipedia.org/wiki/Miller_Reese_Hutchison. Accessed January 20.

https://www.asha.org/about/history/. Accessed January 20.

https://www.english.upenn.edu/sites/www.english.upenn.edu/files/Mills-Mara_Deaf-Jam-Inscription-Reproduction-Information.pdf). Accessed January 20.

Indian Speech & Hearing Association retrieved from http://www.ishaindia. org.in/pdf/Scope_of_Practice.pdf. Accessed January 20.

Ingeborg Hochmair. 2013. *"Vorzeigeunternehmerin mit Berufung." (in German). APA-Science. 12 September 2013.*

Irwin, F. 1943. "Edwin Burket Twitmyer: 1873-1943." *American Journal of Psychology*, 56, 451-453.

Itard, J. M. G. 1962. *The wild boy of Aveyron*. Translated by G. Humphrey & M. Humphrey. New York: Appleton-Century-Crofts. (Original was published in 1801).

J. Eisenson (Ed.), 1958. *Stuttering: A symposium*. 121–166. New York: Harper.

James Sonnett Greene. 1880-1950. Retrieved from https://www.acsu.buffalo.edu/~duchan/biographies.html. Accessed January 20.

Jean Marc Gaspard Itard. 1775-1838. Retrieved from http://www.acsu.buffalo.edu/~duchan/new_history/enlightenment/itard.html. Accessed January 20.

Jewett, D. L., and Williston, J. S. 1971. "Auditory-evoked far fields averaged from the scalp of humans." *Brain*, 94(4):681-96.

Kemp, D. T. 1978. "Stimulated acoustic emissions from within the human auditory system." *J. Acoust. Soc. Amer.* 64 (5): 1386.

Kester, D. 1950. *The development of speech correction in organizations and in schools in the United States during the first quarter of the twentieth century*. PhD diss., Northwestern University. Retrieved from http://www.acsu.buffalo.edu/~duchan/new_history/enlighten ment/sheridan.html. Accessed January 20.

Klatt, D. 1987. "Review of text-to-speech conversion for English." *J. Acoust. Soc. Amer.* 82 (3): 737–93. doi:10.1121/1.395275.

Klingbeil, G.M. 1939. "The historical background of the modern speech clinic. "Journal *of Speech Disorders, 4*, 115-132.

Kucera, Henry. 1983. "Roman Jakobson." *Language: Journal of the Linguistic Society of America* 59(4): 871–883.

Liberman, A. M., Ingemann, F., Lisker, L., Delattre, P. C., and Cooper, F. S. "Minimal rules for synthesizing speech." *J. Acoust. Soc. Amer.*, 1959, 31, 1490-1499.

MacLeod, Elizabeth. 1999. *Alexander Graham Bell: An Inventive Life*. Toronto, Ontario: Kids Can Press. p. 19. ISBN 978-1-55074-456-9.

Introduction to Speech-Language Pathology and Audiology   241

Mahabharata (Ve:davya:sa, Dwapara yuga). 1967. Edited by T. R. Krishnacharya & T. R. Vyasacarya Nirnayasagara Press. Bombay. 12-320-91 to 92.

Mark Aronoff, Janie Rees-Miller (Eds.). 2008. *The Handbook of Linguistics*, John Wiley & Sons, p. 96.

Martin, V. 2007. *History of Speech Language Pathology and Audiology in Canada: Our First Fifty Years.* Winnipeg, Manitoba: Virginia Martin. ISBN 978-0-9783046-0-7.

Max Wien 1903. Retrieved from https://en.wikipedia.org/wiki/ Audiometry. Accessed January 20.

McCarthy, D. 1929. "A comparison of children's language in different situations and its relation to personality traits. "Journal *of Genetic Psychology*, 36. 583-591.

McGinnis, M. 1929. "Diagnosis of congenital aphasia and word-deaf mutes." *Oralism and Auralism*, 8, 35-38.

Menzies, R. G., Onslow, M., and Packman, A. 1999. "Anxiety and stuttering: Exploring a complex relationship." *Journal of Speech, Language, and Hearing Research*, 51, 1451–1464.

Mercurialis, Hieronymus. 1583/1977. "Treatises on the diseases of children." *Journal of Communication Disorders*, 10, 127-140. (Tr, J Wollock).

Mercurialis, Hieronymus. 1659/1977. *de Arte Gymnastica*. Translated by Johannes Chosczieyoioskius and J Wollock, *Journal of Communication Disorders*, 10, 127-140.

Meyer-Eppler, W. 1953. "Zum Erzeugungsmechanismus des Gerauschlaute," *Z. fiir Phonetik* 314, 196-212.

Mills, Mara. 2011. "Hearing Aids and the History of Electronics Miniaturization." *IEEE Annals of the History of Computing.* 33 (2): 24. doi:10.1109/MAHC.2011.43.

Moore, P., and Kester, D. 1953. "Historical notes on speech correction in the pre-association era." *Journal of Speech and Hearing Disorders*, 18, 48-53.

242 *S. R. Savithri*

Moses Mendelssohn. 1729-1786. Retrieved from https://www.acsu. buffalo.edu/~duchan/new_history/enlightenment/enlightenment_disa bility.html. Accessed January 20.

Mudry, A., and Mills, M. 2013. "The early history of the cochlear implant: a retrospective." *JAMA otolaryngology - head & neck surgery.* 139 (5): 446–53.

Mursilis. 1344 – 1320. Retrieved from http://www.acsu.buffalo. edu/~duchan/new_history/ancient_history/mesopotamia.html. Accessed January 20.

Newby, H. A., and Popelka, G. R. 1992. *Audiology* (6th Ed). New Jersey: A Simon & Schuster Company.

Notker Balbulus. 1969. *Charlemagne, in Two Lives of Charlemagne.* In Lewis Thorpe (Harmondsworth (Ed.). A gossipy life of Charlemagne, written by Notker.

Ondrejovic, S. 1996. *Wolfgang von Kempelen and his Mechanism of human speech.* Retrieved from http://www.ling.su.se/staff/hartmut/cache/ ondr_en.htm. Accessed January 20.

O'Neill, Y. V. 1980. *Speech and speech disorders in Western Thought before 1600.* Westport, CO: Greenwood Press.

Orton, S. 1925. "Word blindness in school children." *Archives of Neurology and Psychiatry*, 14, 581-615.

Oza, R. K. 1966. Retrieved from http://www.tnmcnair.com/depts/ast1.html. Accessed January 20.

Paden, E. 1970. *A history of the American Speech and Hearing Association.* Washington, D. C.: The American Speech and Hearing Association.

Palmer, M. F. 1963. Retrieved from https://www.kansas.com/opinion/opn-columns-blogs/article199371554.html. Accessed January 20.

Potter, R. K., Kopp, G. A., and Green, H. C. 1947. *Visible Speech.* New York: Van Nostrand.

Raphael, L. J., Bordon, G. J., and Harris, K. S. 2006. *Speech Science Primer: Physiology, Acoustics, and Perception of Speech.* (6th Ed.). Lippincott: Williams and Wilkins.

Ratna, N. 1965. Retrieved from records of the Institute of Logopedics, Mysore. Accessed January 20.2017.

Introduction to Speech-Language Pathology and Audiology   243

Raymond Carhart. 1912-1975. *Papers, 1938-1975.* Northwestern University Archives, Evanston, Illinois. http://files.library. northwestern.edu/findingaids/raymond_carhart.pdf Accessed 2006-07-31. Accessed January 20.

Raymond Herbert Stetson. 1951. *Motor phonetics: A study of speech movements in action.* Amsterdam: North-Holland Pub. Co.

Rieber, R. W., and Brubeker, R. S. 1966. *Speech Pathology: An international study of science.* Amsterdam: North-Holland Publishing Company.

Rieber, R. W., and Wollock, J. 1977. "The historical roots of the theory and therapy of stuttering." *Journal of Communication Disorders*, 10, 3-24.

Riley, G. D. 1972. "A Stuttering Severity Instrument for Children and Adults. "Journal *of Speech and Hearing Disorders,* 37, 3, 314 – 322. https://doi.org/10.1044/jshd.3703.314.

Robert, B., and Deborah, J. W., (Eds.). 1998. *Instruments of Science: An Historical Encyclopedia.* The Science Museum, London and the National Museum of American History, Smithsonian Institution in Association with Garland Publishing Inc. New York and London: A Member of Taylor and Francis Group.

Rockey, D. 1979. "John Thelwall and the origins of British speech therapy." *Medical History,* 23, 156-175.

Rudolph Agricola. 1444 - 1485. Retrieved from http://www.acsu. buffalo.edu/~duchan/new_history/middle_ages/major_players.html. Accessed January 20.

Russell, G. O., and Tuttle, C. H. 1930. "Colour movies of vocal cord action – an aid in diagnosis." *Laryngoscope,* 40, 549-552.

Sastri, H. Chatterjee, (Ed.).1977. *The Philosophy of Nāgārjuna as contained in the Ratnāvalī.* Part I (Containing the text and introduction only). Saraswat Library, Calcutta.

Saussure, Ferdinand de. 1983. *Course in General Linguistics.* Charles Bally and Albert Sechehaye (Eds.). Translated by Roy Harris. La Salle, Illinois: Open Court. ISBN 0-8126-9023-0.

Savithri, S. R. 1987. "Speech pathology in Ancient India - A review of Sanskrit literature." *Journal of Communication Disorders,* 20(6), 1987 437-445.

Schaefer, K. L., Gruschke, G., Griessmann, B., and Schwarzkopf, H. 1919. Retrieved from https://en.wikipedia.org/wiki/Audiometry. Accessed January 20.

Scheerenberger, R. C. 1983. *History of mental retardation.* Baltimore: Paul H. Brookes.

Schroeder, J. 2000. "Nagarjuna. Upa:ya kausaya hr.daya." *Phylosophy East and West.* Vol. 50, 4.

Scripture, E. W. 1902. *The elements of experimental phonetics.* New York: Scribner and Sons.

Seashore, C. E. 1899. Retrieved from https://en.wikipedia.org/wiki/ Audiometry. Accessed January 20.

Seguin, E. 1866. Retrieved from http://www.disabilityhistorywiki.org/ wiki/index.php?title=Edward_Seguin. Accessed January 20.

Seguin, E. 1866-1971. *Idiocy and its treatment by the physiological method.* New York: A. M. Kelley.

Shipley, K. G., and McAfer, J. G. 2004. *Assessment in Speech-Language Pathology – A Resource manual.* (4th Ed.). Delmar: Cengage Learning.

Silman, S., and Emmer, M. B. 2012. *Instrumentation for Audiology and Hearing Science.* USA: McNaughton and Gunn.

Simmons, F. B., and Smith, W. 1966. "The teacher in Puritan culture." *Harvard Educational Review,* 36, 394-411.

Simmons, F. B., and White, R. J. 1964. Cited by A. Mudry, & Mara Mills in "The Early History of the Cochlear Implant: A Retrospective." *JAMA Otolaryngol Head Neck Surg.* 2013;139(5):446-453.

Simmons, F. B., Mongeon, C. J., Lewis, W. R., and Huntington, D. A. 1964. "Electrical stimulation of acoustic nerve and inferior colliculus." *Arch Otolaryngol.*79:29. 559-68.

Siraisi, N. 1985. "Pietro d'Abano and Taddeo Alderotti: Two Models of Medical Culture." *Medioevo,* 11,139-162.

Introduction to Speech-Language Pathology and Audiology 245

Sohmer, H., and Feinmesser, M. 1967. Cited by Hall, James W. 2007. *New handbook of auditory evoked responses*. Boston: Pearson. ISBN 978-0-205-36104-5. OCLC 71369649.

Soranus of Ephesus. 98 – 138 A D. Retrieved from http://www.acsu.buffalo.edu/~duchan/new_history/ancient_history/major_players.html. Accessed January 20.

Sutton, S., Braren, M., and Zubin, J., & John, E. R. 1965. "Evoked-potential correlates of stimulus uncertainty." *Science,* 150 (3700):1187-8.

Sweet, H., 1988. In *Who Was Who 1897–1915*. London: A. & C. Black.

Swift, W. B. 1869 – 1942. Retrieved from http://www.acsu.buffalo.edu/~duchan/new_history/hist19c/subpages/swift.html. Accessed January 20.

Terkildsen, K. 1964. "Clinical Application of Impedance Measurements with a Fixed Frequency Technique." *International Audiology*, Vol. 3 (2), 147-155.

Terkildsen, K. 1964. Retrieved from https://hearinghealthmatters.org/waynesworld/2014/history-acoustic-impedance-measurement/. Accessed January 20.

Thelwall, J. 1805. *Mr. Thelwall's introductory discourse on the nature and objects of elocutionary science and the studies and accomplishments connected with the cultivation of the faculty of oral expression with outlines of a course of lectures on the science and practice of Elocution*. London: Ponterfact. Retrieved from http://www.acsu.buffalo.edu/~duchan/new_history/thelwall/general_bibliography_thelwall.html. Accessed January 20.

Thelwall, J. 1810a. *A letter to Henry Cline. Esq. on imperfect development of the faculties mental and moral as well as constitutional and organic and on the treatment of impediments of speech*. London: Richard Taylor & Co.

Thelwall, R. 1981. The phonetic theory of John Thelwall 1764-1834. Cited in R. E. Asher & Eugenie J. A. Henderson (Eds.). *Towards a history of phonetics*. 186-203. Edinburgh, Scotland: Edinburgh University Press.

246   *S. R. Savithri*

Travis, L. E. 1896 – 1987. Retrieved from https://ashaarchives.omeka.net/exhibits/show/founding/travis. Accessed January 20.

United Nations Convention on Rights of Persons with disabilities. 2006. Retrieved from https://www.un.org/development/desa/disabilities/convention-on-the-rights-of-persons-with-disabilities.html. Accessed January 20.

van der Lely, H. K. 2005. "Domain-specific cognitive systems: insight from Grammatical-SLI." *Trends Cogn. Sci. (Regul. Ed.).* 9 (2): 53–9. PMID 15668097. doi:10.1016/j.tics.2004.12.002.

Van Riper, C. 1969. *Speech correction: Principles and methods.* (4th Ed.). New York: Prentice Hall.

Webb, W. G., and Adler, R. K. 2008. *Neurology for the speech-language pathologist* (5th Ed.). St. Louis, Mo: Mosby/Elsevier.

Werner, E. S. 1850 – 1919. *The Voice.* Retrieved from http://www.acsu.buffalo.edu/~duchan/new_history/hist19c/subpages/werner.html.Edward Lee Accessed January 20.

Wernicke, C. 1848 – 1905. Retrieved from https://en.wikipedia.org/wiki/Carl_Wernicke. Accessed January 20.

West, R. 1892-1968. Retrieved from http://www.acsu.buffalo.edu/~duchan/history_summary.html. Accessed January 20.

Wien, M. 1903. Retrieved from https://en.wikipedia.org/wiki/Audiometry. Accessed January 20.

Wolfgang von Kempelen. 179. *Mechanismus der menschlichen Sprache nebst Beschreibung einer sprechenden Maschine* and *Le Méchanisme de la parole, suivi de la description d'une machine parlante,* Vienna: J.V. Degen. A reprint of the German edition, with an introduction by Herbert E. Brekle and Wolfgang Wildgren (1970), Stuttgart: Frommann-Holzboog. There are also more recent translations into Hungarian and Slovak.

Wolke, H. 1802. Cited by H. Feldmann, in "History of instrumental measuring of hearing acuity: the first acumeter." *Erratum in Laryngorhinootologie.* 1992, 71(12), 658.

Introduction to Speech-Language Pathology and Audiology   247

Wollock, J. 1990. "Communication disorder in renaissance Italy: An unreported case analysis by Hieronymus Mercurialis." *Journal of Communication Disorders*, 23, 1-30.

World Health Organization. 2001. Retrieved from https://www.who.int/classifications/icf/en/. Accessed January 20.

Worthington, Ian. 2000. *Demosthenes: Statesman and Orator*: London & New York: Routledge.

ABOUT THE AUTHOR

S. R. Savithri, PhD

Former Director,
All India Institute of Speech & Hearing, Manasagangothri,
Mysore, Karnataka, India
Email: alamelu1080@gmail.com

Dr. S. R. Savithri completed her BSc (Speech & Hearing), MSc (Speech & Hearing), and PhD (Speech & Hearing) from the All India Institute of Speech & Hearing, Mysore, affiliated to the University of Mysore. She started her carrier as Research Assistant at the All India Institute of Speech & Hearing, Mysore in the year 1981, then became a faculty in 1986 and finally reached the topmost position of Director of the Institute which is under the Ministry of Health & Family Welfare, Govt. of India. She has over 140 publications in national and international journals and has edited several books and journals. She has received several awards including Sir. C. V. Raman's award for the best paper published in the Journal of the Acoustical Society of India, Sir. M. Visweswaraiah award as a woman scientist and several oration awards. Dr. Savithri retired in July, 2017 as Director upon superannuation. However, the Govt. of India reappointed her for another year as Director and she superannuated in October, 2018.

INDEX OF NAMES

A

Aesop, 202, 234
Agricola, Rudolph, 202, 243
Albertus Magnus, 202, 235
Anon, 196, 235
ANSI S1.1-1994, 58, 139
Aristotle, 202, 235

B

Baken, R. J., 142, 154, 217, 235
Balbulus, 202, 242
Ballantyne, A., 34, 47, 236
Barry, T., 182, 185
Bell, Alexander Graham, 147, 197, 198, 210, 213, 240
Bell, Alexander Melville, 210
Beranek, L. L., 176, 185
Berger, H., 219, 238
Bhartṛhari, 190, 207
Blanton, S., 196, 235
Bloomfield, L., 207, 235
Bode, H. W., 221, 235
Bomar, J. M., 139, 238

Bordon, G J., 140, 242
Borst, J. M., 236
Braren, M., 219, 245
Broca, P., 51, 119, 140, 197, 198, 237
Brodmann, Korbinian, xv, 117, 118, 139, 238
Brogden, W. J., 176, 185

C

Caelius Aurelianus, 202, 236
Canfield, Norton, 186, 194
Caraka, 113, 236
Carhart, R., 194, 243
Ceponiene, R., 34, 47, 236
Churcher, B. G., 178, 185
Clark, Graeme , 222, 238
Clark, J. G., 186, 222, 236
Claudius, 202, 236
Cleave, P.L., 47
Comstock, A., 197, 236
Conti-Ramsden, 34, 47
Cooley, C. H., 112, 139
Cooper, F., 214, 236, 240
Coppola, G., 139, 238
Crichton, A., 191, 237

252   *Index of Names*

Crystal, David, 37, 47
Cummings, A., 34, 47, 236

D

Damasio, A., 119, 139, 237
Darwin, C., 197
Darwin, E., 191
Davis, Hallowell, 219, 237
Davis, Pauline, 219
Delattre, Pierre, 214, 236, 240
Demosthenes, 202, 247
Duchan, J., 237
Dudley, H. W., 213, 239
Duffy, J. R., 129, 139

E

Emmer, M. B., 220, 244
Eustacia, 202, 237

F

Fant, G., 89, 90, 91, 94, 97, 105, 108, 139
Farr, B., 38, 48
Fastl, H., 180, 185
Feinmesser, M., 221, 245
Fletcher, H., 178, 185, 220, 237
Fourcin, A., 217, 237
Fowler, E. P., 220, 237
Franklin, B., 191, 192, 214, 235

G

Gao, F., 139, 238
Garcia, Manual Patricia Rodriguez, 216
Gelfand, S. A., 167, 168, 169, 170, 171,
   173, 174, 175, 185, 238
Gelgic, 34, 47
Geschwind, D. H., 137, 139, 238

Gesner, J. A. P., 191, 238
Greene, E. B., 238
Greene, J. S., 197, 240
Griessmann, B., 220, 244
Gruschke, G., 220, 244

H

Hänsler, H., 179, 185
Harris, K S., 140, 242, 243
Hartmann, W. M, 177, 185, 187
Helmholtz, Herman Ludwig Ferdinand von,
   209
Herman, I. P., 185
Hertz, Heinrich Rudolf, 238
Hirsh, I. J., 185
Hittite king, Mursilis, 202, 242
Hochmair, I., 222, 239
Hosford-Dunn, H., 146, 155
House, W. F., 222, 239

I

Isabel, R., 201
Itard, J. M. G., 192, 203, 240

J

Jakobson, R., 207, 240
Jewett, D. L., 221, 240
John, E. R., 245
Johnson, K., 186
Jonsson, Z. O., 139, 238

K

Kemp, D. T., 221, 240
King, A. J., 185
Konopka, G., 137, 139, 238
Kopp, G. A., 242

Index of Names

L

Ladefoged, P., 140
Landau, L. D., 143, 155
Levitt, H., 169, 173, 174, 186
Liberman, A. M., 214, 236, 240
Lifchitz, E. M., 143, 155
Lum, J. A., 34, 47

M

MaGinnis, Mildred, 197
McCarthy, Dorothea, 198
Mendelssohn, M., 191, 242
Mercurialis, Hieronymous, 202
Meyer-Eppler, W., 97, 140, 241
Miller, G. A., 185
Moore, B. C. J., 186
Moore, P., 241
Muckey, Floyd Summer, 198, 237
Munson, W. A., 185

N

Nagarjuna, Bodhisattva, 113, 140, 244
Nave, C. R., 149, 186
Newby, H. A., 186, 193, 199, 200, 201, 242
Nieto, S., 38, 47

O

Orlikoff, R. F., 142, 154, 235
Orton, S. T., 197, 198, 242
Oza, Ramesh K., 194, 242

P

Pa:ṇini, 207
Palmer, M. F., 194, 242
Palmer, Martin F., 194, 242

Peng, S., 139, 238
Pete, J. R., 186
Peter of Abano, 202
Pierpont, E. I., 34, 48
Popelka, G. R., 186, 193, 199, 200, 201, 242
Potter, R. K., 214, 242
Preuss, T. M., 139, 238

R

Raphael, L. J., 140, 242
Ratna, Natesh, 194, 242
Revesz, G., 136, 139, 238
Rice, M. L., 34, 47
Rieber, R. W., 191, 243
Roeser, R., 146, 155
Rousselot, L'Abbe, 212
Rudmose, W., 176, 187
Russell, George Oscar, 198

S

Saussure, Ferdinand de, 36, 207, 243
Schaefer, K. L., 220, 244
Scheerenberger, R. C., 192, 244
Schmidt, G., 179, 185
Schwarzkopf, H., 220, 244
Scripture, E. W., 197, 244
Seashore, Carl Emil, 198, 220, 236, 244
Seguin, E., 192, 244
Silman, S., 220, 244
Simmons, F. B., 222, 244
Sivian, L. J., 176, 187
Sohmer, H., 221, 245
Soranus of Ephesus, 202, 245
Starkweather, C. W., 14, 48
Stetson, Raymond Herbert, 212, 243
Stevens, S. S., 177, 179, 187
Sutton, S., 219, 245
Sweet, Henry, 209
Swift, W. B., 196, 245

254   *Index of Names*

T

Tallal, P., 34, 48
Tampas, J. W., 184, 186
Terkildsen, K., 221, 245
Thelwall, J., 192, 237, 243, 245
Townsend, J., 34, 47, 236
Travis, L. E., 140, 197, 198, 246
Trumbull, E., 38, 48
Tucker, F. M., 184, 186
Twitmyer, E. B., 196, 240

U

Ullman, M.T., 34, 48

V

Valente, M. V., 146, 155
van der Lely, H. K., 34, 48, 246
Van Riper, C., 198, 246
von Békésy, Georg, 221, 238

W

Watson, C. S., 173, 185
Werner, E. S., 193, 196, 246
Wernicke, Carl, 198
Wexler, K., 34, 47
White, R. J., 176, 187, 222, 244
White, Robert, J. , 176, 187, 222, 244
White, S. D., 176, 187, 222, 244
Wien, M., 220, 241, 246
Wien, Max , 220, 241, 246
Winden, K., 139, 238
Wohlschlegel, J. A., 139
Wolke, H., 220, 246
Wollock, J., 191, 241, 243, 247
Wulfeck, B., 34, 47, 236

Z

Zubin, J., 219, 245
Zwicker, E., 180, 185

INDEX OF TERMS

A

action potential, 114, 115, 164
alphabet, 209, 210
alveolar ridge, 7, 8, 197
alveolus, 6, 7
aphasia, 118, 119, 120, 121, 123, 127, 191, 200, 239, 241
aphonia, 132, 204
apraxia, 33, 119, 120
articulation, xv, 3, 5, 6, 7, 8, 9, 12, 14, 24, 25, 46, 91, 96, 105, 112, 128, 132, 191, 197, 200, 202, 204, 207, 208, 210, 217
auditory cortex, 120, 132
auditory nerve, 131, 132, 164
autonomic nervous system, 117, 134, 138

B

babbling, 25, 26, 28, 137
background noise, 184, 186
basal ganglia, 116, 117, 122, 129, 134
basilar membrane, 158, 162, 164, 165
Bordon, G J., 140, 242

brain, 14, 23, 33, 50, 51, 58, 114, 115, 117, 118, 119, 120, 121, 123, 125, 126, 137, 158, 162, 165, 197, 205, 219, 221, 236
brain damage, 33, 127
brain functioning, 219
brainstem, 116, 117, 123, 127, 129, 138, 158, 162, 166, 221
breathing, 22, 31, 53, 134, 179

C

central nervous system (CNS), 50, 116, 158, 165, 233
cerebellum, xv, 117, 122, 123, 127, 138
cerebral cortex, 116, 117, 118, 122, 129, 158, 162, 165
cerebral hemisphere, xii, xv, 52, 117, 118, 120, 121, 123
cerebral palsy, 34, 202, 205
cerebrospinal fluid, 125, 126
cerebrum, xv, 117, 120, 121, 122
cleft lip, 205
cleft palate, 34, 200, 205, 227
cochlea, xv, 51, 132, 133, 158, 161, 162, 163, 164, 221, 222

256 *Index of Terms*

cochlear implant, 190, 206, 222, 228, 232, 236, 242

communication, 1, 2, 15, 19, 20, 21, 23, 28, 33, 38, 46, 111, 136, 192, 195, 202, 204, 205, 224, 225, 226, 227, 229, 230, 231, 232

communication skills, 38, 226, 227

communication systems, 227

cortex, 116, 117, 118, 119, 120, 122, 123, 124, 127, 129, 130, 131, 133

cranial nerve, xv, 51, 123, 128, 129, 130, 131, 133, 166, 228, 233

cranium, 51, 125

D

decibel, vii, 141, 143, 146, 147, 148, 149, 150, 151, 152, 153, 154, 170, 181

disability, 196, 222, 230, 232, 242

dysarthria, 34, 119, 122, 123, 129, 130

E

echolalia, 29, 30, 31

education, 15, 19, 35, 38, 44, 192, 194, 196, 205, 224, 226, 229, 231, 233, 234, 237

educational programs, 192, 201, 229

F

facial expression, 20, 21, 132

frontal lobe, 21, 51, 118, 119, 127

G

genes, 137, 139, 238

genetic disorders, 227

genetics, 49

google, 24, 54, 59, 90, 106, 107, 124, 172

H

habituation, 170, 172

hair cells, 158, 162, 164, 165

health care professionals, 205, 223

hearing impairment, 24, 33, 178, 182, 214, 227, 229, 233

hearing loss, 24, 33, 186, 205, 206, 221, 228, 230, 233

history, 35, 38, 43, 45, 137, 190, 197, 198, 217, 234, 235, 236, 237, 238, 239, 240, 242, 243, 245, 246

Hittite king, Mursilis, 202, 242

Hochmair, I., 222, 239

human brain, 137, 178, 219

hypothalamus, 116, 123, 134

I

IASP, 182, 185

impulses, 14, 21, 113, 114, 115, 130, 131, 133, 136, 164

inner ear, 23, 133, 157, 159, 161, 162, 164, 165, 166, 221

intracranial pressure, 126

ipsilateral, 128, 129

L

language development, vii, 27, 33, 35, 46

language impairment, 33, 47, 48, 236

language processing, 204

language proficiency, 227

languages, 9, 10, 11, 12, 14, 34, 35, 36, 37, 38, 39, 40, 41, 42, 43, 44, 45, 46, 47, 195, 202, 207, 223

laryngectomy, 227

laryngoscope, 216, 217

larynx, 3, 6, 8, 22, 51, 52, 54, 55, 89, 92, 119, 137, 217

Index of Terms

M

medicine, 193, 196, 198, 200, 209, 215
medulla, 116, 122, 123, 127, 128, 130, 131
medulla oblongata, 123
mental retardation, 33, 192, 205, 244
motor actions, 51
motor activity, 119
motor behavior, 25, 122
motor control, 25, 123
motor neurons, 123, 138
motor system, 129, 130
movement disorders, 129
music, 39, 93, 182, 214

N

nasopharynx, 8, 157, 161
nervous system, 21, 33, 49, 50, 51, 52, 89, 114, 117, 123, 125, 127, 133, 134, 136, 138
nervousness, 134
neurotransmitter(s), 114, 115, 116, 123, 138

O

occipital lobe, 51, 118, 120, 122, 127, 133
optic chiasm, 133
optic nerve, 133
oral cavity, 1, 5, 6, 7, 23, 55, 89, 96, 104, 108, 109
ossicles, 157, 161, 163, 165, 178

P

palate, 6, 7, 8, 10, 12, 51, 56, 57, 107, 119, 197, 205, 217
parasympathetic nervous system, 50, 117
parietal lobe, 51, 119, 127, 133
pharynx, 6, 7, 8, 9, 23, 51, 55, 104, 161

phonemes, ix, 16, 25, 28, 30, 31, 34, 207, 208, 213
phonology, 16, 19, 27, 46, 204, 211
pitch, xi, 4, 15, 30, 68, 71, 131, 132, 204
primary function, 22, 23, 56
primary visual cortex, 120, 133

R

reading, 119, 120, 133, 191, 197, 199, 201, 203, 227, 229, 234
reading comprehension, 119, 120, 133, 227
rehabilitation, 193, 199, 201, 203, 228, 229, 232
repetitions, 14, 26, 30, 32, 79
resonator, xv, xvi, 57, 97, 106, 110, 111, 160, 190, 208, 209
respiration, 8, 22, 23, 53, 128, 130, 131, 136
response, xiii, 20, 85, 100, 112, 124, 167, 168, 170, 173, 174, 176, 178, 179, 181, 219, 220, 221
rhythm, 15, 204
right hemisphere, 118, 119

S

sensation, 50, 58, 61, 63, 117, 123, 181, 203, 209, 239
sensitivity, 152, 154, 165, 168, 220
sensorineural hearing loss, 183
serotonin, 115, 116
signals, 19, 20, 50, 115, 117, 149, 152, 158, 165, 180, 187, 215, 217, 222
signs, 19, 20
sine wave, xii, 67, 68, 69, 70, 75, 79, 80, 138, 178, 180
skeletal muscle, 157, 161, 215
speech perception, 23, 190, 207, 214
speech sounds, 5, 6, 9, 10, 11, 12, 13, 14, 16, 23, 26, 28, 34, 46, 57, 84, 88, 99, 111, 119, 190, 198, 210, 214

258 *Index of Terms*

spinal cord, xv, 50, 51, 116, 117, 122, 123, 124, 125, 126, 127, 129, 130, 131, 133, 166, 233

stimulation, 33, 34, 49, 164, 165, 244

stimulus, 19, 115, 158, 165, 166, 167, 168, 169, 170, 171, 172, 173, 174, 178, 182, 221, 245

T

teachers, 48, 192, 193, 199, 210

techniques, 173, 176, 193, 197, 216

technological advances, 221

technology, 154

teeth, 2, 5, 7, 8, 56, 97

telephone, 19, 210, 220, 222

temporal lobe, 51, 120, 127, 134, 158, 162

thalamus, 116, 117, 123, 131, 133

therapy, 191, 192, 194, 198, 204, 205, 211, 243

tinnitus, 228, 229

tones, 55, 68, 71, 88, 97, 159, 167, 175, 177, 181, 187, 209, 210

trachea, 1, 8, 21, 22, 52, 54

training, 27, 192, 193, 198, 199, 200, 201, 202, 223, 224, 227, 231, 233

training programs, 223, 231

transmission, 23, 75, 113, 114, 116, 154, 163, 213

treatment, 89, 191, 202, 204, 205, 206, 231, 244, 245

tympanic membrane, 157, 159, 161, 163, 221

tympanometry, 221

U

utricle, 162, 166

uvula, 7, 9

V

vibration, xiii, 3, 4, 14, 49, 55, 57, 58, 60, 61, 63, 67, 68, 70, 71, 72, 78, 80, 82, 83, 84, 85, 86, 93, 94, 101, 123, 138, 158, 160, 163, 165, 166

viscera, 51, 131

vision, 120, 123, 133, 192

visual stimuli, 120

visual system, 133

vocabulary, 28, 29, 30, 31, 32, 33, 35, 37, 39, 40, 135

vocalizations, 211

voicing, 13, 14, 22, 102

W

word blindness, 197

Related Nova Publications

COMMUNICATIONS: GOVERNMENT POLICIES AND PROGRAMS

AUTHOR: Tatum Mangum

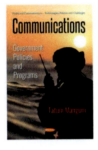

SERIES: Media and Communications – Technologies, Policies and Challenges

BOOK DESCRIPTION: The WIN-T program is the Army's high-speed, high-capacity tactical communications network to distribute classified and unclassified information through all echelons of Army command by means of voice, data and real-time video.

SOFTCOVER ISBN: 978-1-53614-200-6
RETAIL PRICE: $82

COMMUNICATIONS AND NETWORKING: PERSPECTIVES, OPPORTUNITIES AND CHALLENGES

EDITOR: Geng Liang

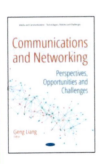

SERIES: Media and Communications – Technologies, Policies and Challenges

BOOK DESCRIPTION: This book provides a comprehensive study on how to use networks to support industrial communication application.

HARDCOVER ISBN: 978-1-53613-858-0
RETAIL PRICE: $230

To see a complete list of Nova publications, please visit our website at www.novapublishers.com